WHAT I GOT INSTEAD

A Story of Pain,
Doubt, and Faith

EILEEN F. SOMMI

HIGH BRIDGE BOOKS

What I Got Instead
by Eileen F. Sommi

Printed in the United States of America
ISBN (Paperback): 978-1-954943-90-2
ISBN (Hardcover): 978-1-962802-01-7

This work depicts actual events in the life of the author as truthfully as recollection permits and/or can be verified by research. Occasionally, dialogue consistent with the character or nature of the person speaking has been supplemented. All persons within are actual individuals; there are no composite characters. The names of some individuals have been changed to respect their privacy.

High Bridge Books titles may be purchased in bulk for educational, business, fundraising, or sales promotional use. For information, please contact High Bridge Books via www.HighBridgeBooks.com/contact.

Published in Houston, Texas, by High Bridge Books

To Mike Sommi

My life and this book wouldn't be what it is without you.
I am beyond grateful for your steadfast love,
kindness, faithfulness, and endless support.
Yours truly and always.

To Denise DeRosa

Our friendship is woven into the pages of this book.
I couldn't have endured the writing of it without
your constant support and encouragement.

To Jo Kadlecek

Without you, I would never have written a word.

To Robyn and Bruce Wagner

My prayer warriors and friends,
thank you for helping me get over this finish line.

To My Children

Matt, Cole, Kit, and Grace
You continue to give me endless joy and a
life worth fighting for. Gosh, I love you guys.

Contents

Introduction

If there is meaning in life at all, then there must be meaning in suffering.

—Viktor Frankl[1]

IT HURTS. PAIN IS PAIN whether it's throbbing, acute, chronic, occasional, physical, spiritual, emotional, self-inflicted, undeserved, genetic, or psychosomatic. It has no prejudice and every soul past, present, and future will contend with it to some degree. Pain knows no boundaries, has no sympathy, and, apparently, is here to stay.

If I didn't believe in a good God, I wouldn't have such a problem with pain; but, from a young age, I've had trouble coming to terms with a loving God who watches his children suffer—even though he possesses the power to heal and deliver anyone out of their misery. Sometimes he does heal, but oftentimes people suffer and die with their pain unresolved.

It's disturbing.

Because my pain is physical and chronic, I've wrestled with it long enough to get sweaty and sore in the process. Along the way, I've had some victories in understanding pain's purpose and many defeats when facing its relentlessness and severity. Also, because my pain is not life threatening, I've been able to contemplate and write about what I've learned from this unwanted, yet often effective teacher.

So, I will share my story. It is not that my story is any more significant than anyone else's story; it's just that it's not any less. I hope telling my story will help you with yours. Perhaps if I share honestly, you'll do the same. Maybe my wrestling will encourage your wrestling. And, if you are living with pain, maybe reading about someone else living with pain will just be good company.

1

A Million Questions

The master key of knowledge is, indeed, a persistent and frequent questioning.

—Peter Abelard

I REMEMBER ONE PARTICULAR MORNING FEELING ESPECIALLY BAD. Our four kids—Matt, Cole, Kit, and Grace—shuffled around the kitchen getting ready for their Saturday morning activities. Matt was our oldest and soon-to-be thirteen. Cole followed two years behind Matt, and Kit just celebrated her ninth birthday. Grace was our baby at five-and-a-half years old. It was spring and the three oldest kids were involved in one of our family's favorite sports—lacrosse. My husband, Mike, always coached one of the kids' teams, and so every weekend revolved around games and practices.

Living on Long Island where lacrosse is king, you are lucky if it is your sport of choice because there is plenty of it to go around. I never played since our high school didn't have girls' lacrosse, but my husband, Mike, played all the way through college. When our kids took a liking to it, to say Mike was elated would be an understatement. As for me, when I feel good, there is nothing better than a Saturday of lacrosse, but with my head about to explode from the current migraine, I knew I wouldn't be joining them up at the high school. The normal morning prep seemed like chaos. The simplest task was a mountain to climb. I poured milk and buttered bagels, trying to feed everyone before they headed out the door.

I rarely complained to the kids about my migraines. Growing up is challenging enough without your mother complaining about her pain. So, I prepared a simple breakfast without a whisper of my current condition. Grace jumped up on the counter so I could fix her hair, and in the distance, I could hear Matt yelling for his mouth guard which he couldn't find—yet again.

Gosh, his voice is loud.

Kit was packing up her stick and eye goggles while Mike gathered his coaching paraphernalia. Once Grace's hair was finished, I walked to the mudroom to see if I could find Matt's mouthpiece, trying hard not to jostle my head. Rounding the corner, I found sports equipment strewn across the floor. Cole was looking for his elbow pads. I let out an audible groan.

Mike walked in, stepping over Cole and the mess.

"See you later. I hope your head feels better," he said, giving me a hug. "Grace can come with me and help coach the boys, but tell the kids to get out to the truck. We've gotta run."

Spotting Cole's elbow pads under a gym bag, I pointed at the floor, directing him to the missing piece. It's such a relief when the lost are found.

"Thanks, Mom, see you later," Cole said, picking up his stuff and running out the door with a bagel in his cute fist.

"Matt. Girls. Dad is already in the truck. Hurry," I said.

"Kit, do you have everything?" I asked while shoving a water bottle in her bag and kissing her forehead.

"Yup. Thanks, and can I go home with Julia after practice?" Kit asked, heading for the door.

"Ask your father. Have fun and hopefully I'll see you later."

Grace ran past me with a coach's whistle around her neck and Matt right behind her. I watched from the front porch as the Suburban tore out of the driveway. Leaning on one of the porch columns, I took a deep breath and smiled. I was grateful for my family. Crazy how much you love them. I watched them drive down Goose Hill

Road toward the high school fields where all their friends would be waiting. I turned to go back inside, whispering a prayer of thankfulness, and then planted my body along with my aching head on the couch.

I hate being left behind, watching everyone run out the door with a fun day ahead of them. It's not right. Days are meant to be lived, and I had no desire to lie around with my head immobilized, waiting for relief from yet another migraine. My head pounded. I heard the phone ring, but let it go. The breakfast dishes waited. And then the questions I have asked for so long surfaced yet again: Why doesn't God take the pain away? I have literally asked a thousand times over. And not just my pain, everyone's. Could he possibly cause it? Or, does he just allow it? How can he bear to watch? How can he listen to the cries and not do something?

It had been an especially bad week of migraines, and when the pain lasts for days in a row without a break, I am usually thin skinned, temperamental, and weak. I've lost my patience with the whole thing. I want it to be over, and when I wake up with its presence for yet another day, I could crumble. Or scream. This was one of those days.

I often want to argue my condition with someone, and usually no one is around, so it ends up being me and God, which is good since he made me this way. Why don't you help me? Or do you? Are you really who you say you are? Why won't you make my head work in a new way? Maybe you could rewire me? Redirect and restructure my blood vessels? Make my crazy neck muscles relax?

He could do it. But, he hasn't.

So, I figure he must have a purpose for the pain. And, it can't be just to watch me (or you) suffer. So what was it? What did God want from me? Aside from the pounding in my head, I heard nothing. No answers.

My thoughts wandered to the book of Psalms where Israel's King David writes that God has taken account of our wanderings, put our tears in his bottle and in his book.[2] So, if he is keeping track of all this sadness, why won't he just eliminate it? How can he watch his creation suffer? I can't even watch my dog suffer without jumping in to ease *his* pain or pull him from trouble. How can I have more compassion for my dog than God has for human beings?

I can't. That's the point.

As I continued my thought process lying on the couch far from the lacrosse field, it occurred to me that perhaps pain relief wasn't at the top of God's "to-do" list. From my vantage point, he didn't seem remotely interested in pain relief. He seemed to think differently about it than I did. He seemed more comfortable with pain than the rest of us. I don't get it. All I know is it makes me mad.

The sun continued to shine through the French doors in the family room, and I wished I could at least get up and climb the small hill in our backyard to the garden. The beds needed weeding and I loved being on my knees in the dirt. I thought about the lettuce I wanted to plant and the sweet peas. It was still spring and there was plenty of time for my seeds to germinate and be harvested in time. I mulled over the different vegetables I had chosen for this year's planting and daydreamed about the flower seeds that would grow into a delightful array of color from zinnias to cosmos. Who tires of the miracle of planting a tiny seed and watching it sprout and grow into something beautiful and even edible? I know I will never get over it.

I got up to make a hot compress for my head and lied down again with it draped over my eyes and forehead, covering my temples. The heat and darkness felt good. The questions to God did not. So why won't you ease our pain? What would be the harm in it?

"Where are you in our present trouble?" I whimpered.

I wished I could fall asleep, but it was impossible with the pounding going on inside my skull. Maybe I was going down the wrong track. Maybe this world is not under God's jurisdiction, but Satan's—someone I assume would take great pleasure in our pain. I don't spend a lot of time thinking about the devil, but, once in a while, I do. The Bible describes him as someone who is constantly seeking to "destroy" us. "Destroy" is a pretty strong word. It means to obliterate, annihilate, demolish, devastate, raze, or wipe out.[3] So, if Satan does have a say on this earth, some of this could make sense.

I think giving someone migraines and headaches for most of her life is a very clever way to go about trying to destroy her. If this good earth isn't God's kingdom come, the hope is that God is with us here, by our side, to help us endure. Is *this* where a loving God makes a difference—in the enduring? That argument would completely work for me if *no one* ever got healed or saved. But *some* do.

It's no wonder I don't allow my mind to wander down this path very often. It's complicated, and I'm never able to get to the end of the logic. There always seems to be a hole in it. I tried sleeping. The drums in my head were too loud, and not only had the tempo picked up, but also the dynamics. My compress was cold now, so I took it off and covered my head (with one of Matt's jerseys he'd left on the couch) to block the light streaming in from the windows. Somehow, it's sweaty smell was comforting. I took a deep breath.

Maybe some folks are more deserving than others, more "full of faith?" Are others meant to suffer because of the evil they've inflicted on humanity? Is pain punishment? Or, is it just the harsh reality of an imperfect world?

It's so complicated it makes my head spin.

I went upstairs to my bathroom, hoping to find some Tylenol PM that might put me out of my misery and stop the onslaught of unanswerable questions. We didn't have any. I reached in the cabinet for the Excedrin Migraine. The Excedrin contained caffeine, and I was hoping to fall asleep, so I changed my mind and grabbed a couple of Tylenol and Aspirin instead. My brain was on overload between the pounding and perplexing thoughts—and now I was starting to get nauseous. I closed the blinds on the bedroom windows and crawled into bed.

The questions were certainly not helping my migraine dissipate. I forced myself to stop thinking so much. The nausea mounted, and I got the trash can from the bathroom. Back in bed, I clutched it and tried to vomit. Nothing. I dry heaved into the empty can and then curled my body into a tight ball pulling the covers up over my head. My blinds weren't black-out shades, and the light was annoying. I concentrated on the rhythm of my breathing and after a while slipped off to a semi-sleeping state. I was glad the house was empty and quiet for the moment, and I had the luxury of just lying in bed without anyone around to watch me muddle through.

I wish for answers to my questions. I think about the many who have tried to reconcile it all—intelligent philosophers, writers, teachers, and preachers. There have been books on the subject that have allowed me to taste hope and gain understanding. I have listened to brilliant communicators, drinking in their words for insight. But, when my head is pounding and the drilling sensation between my eyeballs ensues for the tenth day, I cannot understand why God won't heal me—no matter how well-written the prose or beautifully explained his purpose. Despite my compulsion to wrangle with God Almighty, I always end up surrendering in my pain—hoping time passes quickly to the hour of relief.

Insight and understanding usually come over time with the gift of hindsight. So, let me start at the beginning.

For my thoughts are not your thoughts, neither are your ways my ways, declares the Lord. For as the heavens are higher than the earth, so are my ways higher than your ways and my thoughts than your thoughts.

Isaiah 55:8–9, ESV

2

The Beginning

As she spoke she lifted her eyes and looked across the Valley and the river to the lovely sunset-lighted peaks of the mountains, then cried out in desperate longing, "Oh, if only I could escape from this Valley…"

—Hannah Hurnard[4]

I'VE HAD THESE HEADACHES FOR AS LONG AS I CAN REMEMBER. Decades now. Over four. They range from mildly annoying to downright debilitating. Mostly, they inhabit the space right behind my nose and eyeballs. Often, they travel to the base of my neck or forehead. Sometimes, they float over to the left or right side of my head, leaving one side perfectly pain free while the other side screams as it darts around like a caged animal. It's a pressure system that pushes against my face, a drilling sensation that digs deep into my sinuses, crazy pockets of dynamic pain shooting around my cerebrum at will—all of which constantly reminds me that something is not right, and at times, makes me want to puke.

I liken the sensation to accidentally smashing your thumb with a hammer or bending down only to come up quickly and smack your head on the corner of a protruding granite countertop. It's like that some days, only worse because the pain doesn't subside in a few minutes. It stays with you for the day, accompanies you to bed, and wakes up with you in the morning. Those of you who suffer head pain know what I'm talking about and, bottom line, it sucks.

As a kid, I mentioned these headaches to my parents and pediatrician. My parents for some reason didn't think much of it. Having grown up in rural Norway back in the 1940's where you only saw a doctor if you were deathly ill or had a broken bone, the thought never occurred to them to take me to a specialist. From the outside looking in, I seemed to be quite healthy.

The annual visit to my pediatrician went something like this:

Once in the examining room, I would jump up on the table and Dr. Broden would stand before me, staring at his clipboard. His heavy, labored breathing filled the room and exhausted me with its rhythm. Eventually, he'd look up and begin his exam. He would quickly glance up my nostrils, peek in my ears, press on my belly, and hammer my knees to check my reflexes (which he always thought were excellent). Between the breathing and the sweat on his pale, balding brow, I thought he might suffer heart failure before the exam was over. He pushed to finish, asking me to jump on the scale, stand on one leg, bend over so he could make sure my spine was straight, and then signal to me to get dressed by pointing at my clothes on the table. And, it was over.

Before leaving, he would ask me if there was anything else I would like him to know.

"Well, there are those nasty headaches still," I reminded him while quickly slipping my shirt back on.

"How often and how bad are they *this* year?"

"Pretty often and pretty bad," I said with my nose crinkled and head cocked trying to evoke some sympathy. The doctor gave a heavy sigh and my mother appeared impatient with her purse on her elbow and car keys in hand.

"Well, you are still growing, and it isn't unusual for kids to get headaches during these years. I'm sure it's just growing pains, Eileen."

I slid off the table to put on my shorts, amazed at how much it hurt to grow. Truly unbelievable what kids had to go through to get big. And, based on my pain, I concluded I would grow up to be the tallest woman with the biggest head in the world. Scary thought. And that was that. Dr. Broden wished me well in school, and I'd say good-bye until next year.

It never occurred to me to question Dr. Broden's opinion. He was a doctor, and as far as I was concerned, a learned professional with infinite knowledge on matters of the body. My parents never asked for another opinion or pushed him to perform extra tests. His explanation seemed logical enough to them and to me. But deep inside I always wondered if he was wrong.

Year after year, I left his office disappointed that I was in for yet another twelve months of "growing pain" and hoped that one day soon I'd be big enough so the growing, along with its pain, would just stop.

Aside from this annual complaint to Dr. Broden, I rarely talked about my headaches. I assumed everyone was growing and, thus, had some sort of pain with which to contend. I learned subconsciously that keeping busy and trying to ignore it was far better than accepting the reality of pain's presence. I think I believed deep down inside that if I acknowledged it, I would make it worse. Living in denial seemed easier.

My denial would kick in before my feet hit the ground in the morning. I would lift the heavy weight off my pillow and refuse to groan or complain to my sister telling me to "hurry or we'll miss the bus!" But her morning perkiness eluded me. I would sit on the edge of my bed and listen to her routine with a mixture of awe and jealousy. Her light-footed scurry back and forth from bedroom to bathroom was nothing short of extraordinary. I couldn't understand how she moved so fast, completely unbothered, as I assumed she felt some of the growing pains I was feeling. It was amazing and often made me feel like I was just not as tough as she was.

Eventually, I'd hoist myself off my bed, throw on my clothes, slump to the bathroom for a good toothbrushing, and run a brush through my long, straight hair. I'd arrive in the kitchen where my parents waited, insisting I eat something before heading out the door to follow my sister (who was long gone) to the bus stop.

I'd trudge up our driveway (trusting BettyAnn would hold the bus for me) while praying for the throbbing to stop and my headache to dissipate. Sometimes it did. Sometimes it didn't. Whether it did or not, by the time I was on the bus, my mind turned to the day ahead—bus ride conversations, practice after school, homework I forgot, tests I would take, and, of course, the drama of relationships. I loved school, and no matter how I felt, when the bus rolled into the school parking lot, I wasn't about to let my stupid head stand between me and some fun.

Somehow, I believed if I defined my problem aloud, it would overtake me and ruin my life. The longer I kept the pain unnamed, the longer I could ignore the fact that it was a part of every week, and, in some way, affecting my mood, thoughts, and actions. In not dignifying it with a title, I kept the headaches from taking center stage—dictating my days and defining my personality. Or so I thought. I fought hard to bury it.

There were days, too many actually, when ignoring the throbbing pressure was impossible and it would win. I would fade away to my room with a hot towel on my face hoping to fall asleep. Lying there, I'd push back the tears pressing on my eyelids, knowing that crying only made it hurt more.

I remember being in junior high school when the kids on the school bus pointed out the dark circles under my eyes that came as a result of my head problem. I was horrified. I began to dread their questions of why I looked so tired. Some even asked if I'd been in a fight and punched in the face. Not the look I was going for at twelve. One morning bus ride, I finally figured out a solution. After yet another dreaded "Do you have a black eye?" question, I decided to go to the school nurse and carry out a plan to cover up my face.

"Good morning, Miss Hannity," I said with a squint.

"What can I do for you this morning?" she responded—seeming friendly enough. I had never been to the nurse's office and didn't know if she was the type who would fall for what I was about to say.

"Well, I am having trouble seeing the blackboard and things are looking pretty fuzzy this year," I said, conjuring up my best acting skills.

"Sounds like you might need glasses. Let's go ahead and try to read the vision chart on the wall," she replied, grabbing my shoulders and gently turning me toward the large poster with letters.

I went ahead and read off the letters, reading some correctly and some not. I turned *t*'s into *f*'s and *e*'s into *o*'s and left her office with a note to my parents explaining that it seemed I needed glasses, and could they please take me to the eye doctor.

By Monday of the next week, I wore glasses. Everything was slightly blurry, but my dark circles were covered up enough so that my classmates stopped asking me if I was tired or bruised. I considered it a victory and didn't care that my 20/20 vision eyeballs were now covered in prescription glasses. Although my solution had an obvious blurry downside, I was satisfied.

These battles I fought alone, although I did have the company of God. I would lie in bed at night, say my prayers—circling the world to remember my extended family from Norway to Alaska. I would then thank him for all the goodness around me—my warm bed, my family, friends, the horses next door, and maybe something great that had happened that day. Then, I would ask for help with whatever overwhelmed me. It could be a test, a fight with my Dad, or whether I'd get a part in the next school play. Finally, before slipping off to sleep I would ask God again. "And, could you please make it go away?" I would just lie there quietly and wait—fully believing God could stop my pain.

But he never did. Eventually, I would fall asleep.

It was natural for me to wrestle with my pain from a perspective of faith. If you don't believe in God, I imagine my approach is frustrating or confusing. I get that. But, I was raised on faith—a belief in a God who was loving and kind. It was part of my every week and permeated the atmosphere of our family home. The downbeat to every measure of my childhood was faith, whether it was Sunday morning church, Sunday evening church, bedtime prayers, morning devotions, the music we played, my parents' example, Wednesday prayer meeting, Friday youth group, or family prayer. There it was. Every day. Always out in front of me.

I knew plenty of kids who grew up in that atmosphere and *didn't* believe in God. I had moments of doubt and unbelief—sometimes I still do, but mostly I found it easy to believe in a Creator. I would read the Bible—from the beautiful Psalms to the crazy Old Testament stories to Jesus' life on Earth—and it rang true for me. Just being outside at the beach or in the woods—wherever, honestly—I saw evidence of God all around me. I knew he was there.

I'll never forget one particular Easter morning. I must have been about ten years old. Our small church had a guest preacher, and he was describing Christ's crucifixion in detail. I was captivated by the details, the pain, and the love of someone laying down their life for me. I always knew I needed someone to save me. Even though I was a pretty good kid, I knew what was inside of me. I knew my propensity for wrongdoing. I remember trying to be kind for a day straight, and I just couldn't do it. Even though I wanted to be good to others, selfishness would win the moment, or my pride would break a run of good behavior. What is up with that? There had to be something in my nature that was stronger than my desire to be good. Something dragging me down. I always knew I needed someone greater than me to save me from myself. Believing in God came easy.

Because God was real for me, I just assumed he saw me, knew my pain, heard my pleas for help, and would eventually save me, not just from my sins but from the hurt. It was in his nature to do so. Saving people is what he did. When he didn't, I assumed it just wasn't time yet. His ways are not our ways. So, I kept waiting and hoping.

When my pain soared, I would tell my parents. But I didn't complain often since they had taught me not to. A lesson I took to the extreme, I suppose. I'm sure my mother and father would have wanted to know when I was having a headache and not just hear about the more extreme migraine. But the thought of constantly complaining to them about something as minor as a headache was impossible.

Let me explain.

My parents grew up overseas in the countryside of Norway, as I mentioned earlier. World War II interrupted their peaceful, rural upbringing, and they suffered under the Germans who invaded their homes and demanded their food—filling their communities with insecurity and uneasiness. Sometimes, they had to hide in the mountains, share their food with enemy soldiers, and occasionally escape to safer ground in the middle of the night. Heck, my parents grew up with outhouses and horses. They made their own butter, knit their own sweaters, wove their own bed sheets, and grew their own potatoes. No kidding. They were the kids who really did walk miles to school in the fair weather and ski to school in the winter. With that information and some of their stoicism knit into my DNA, I knew moaning to them about my chronic pain wasn't happening—especially when I thought my pain was a normal side effect of growing up.

Aside from their history and my interpretation of it, there was also this ever present, invisible and unspoken mystery in our family that I felt, but never understood. With all our family's goodness and joy, there was also a deep sadness and secrecy that I couldn't put my finger on. There seemed to be issues in the shadows that were not to be spoken of or uncovered. I could be wrong, but my gut told me I wasn't. Was it my Dad's underlying grief from leaving home as an eighteen-year-old kid? As an only son leaving the family farm and moving to a foreign country, I can only imagine the guilt and homesickness he felt. I loved and admired my father's emotion—his passion, enthusiasm and strength, but I was uncomfortable with his unabashed tears when he talked about his home and family far away. It made me feel uneasy and sad.

And then there was my Mom. Why was she so silent?

My mother always had this dignity about her that bordered on regal-ness. She was beautiful. Gorgeous blue eyes, perfect bone structure and teeth, and her lips—well, you couldn't help but notice their graceful curve flanked by the subtle dimples of her cheeks. She was kind and giving with a subtle humor that would surprise me in the best way possible. Along with all her incredible qualities, she was unfortunately distant. I could never figure it out. There was some sort of disconnect. I always wanted to know her more—have a closer relationship, but I couldn't ever break through. She was fiercely protective of her three kids, and I knew I was dearly loved, but she wasn't demonstrative in her expression of love. Some people just aren't, but as a child, I often wished she was. This seeming invisible wall around her heart made me think she was hiding something from us that was too hard to talk about. What made her so resolute in her privacy? Was it just her personality, or did something happen to her? I always wondered. I remember questioning her as a young adult—asking her if there was something painful in her past that made her so private. She stared me in the eyes and announced, "My life is a closed book." It gave me the chills, and I knew I would never ask her that question again.

So, there was that.

My father's strong emotion and my mother's privacy were two powerful, underlying forces in my life that made the simple act of sharing pain impossible. I remember morning prayers at the breakfast table that ended in tears as my dad moved into prayers for his family back home in Norway. I would squirm with discomfort as my dad wept while squeezing my mom's hand. Hard to see your father be so vulnerable and broken. My mom would sit next to him and hold his hand. She would rarely shed a tear and she never offered a prayer. Instead of joining my father in his emotion, I would follow my mother's lead and bite my lip. My dad's unbridled expression of sadness scared me. Her silence, though mysterious, was safer. The prayer would end, and we would clean up the breakfast dishes without a word.

I love my parents. I love their uniqueness and individual flare. My mom's quiet grace and dignity and my dad's love and energy were beyond compare. I know they raised us in the best way they knew, and I will be forever grateful. Now that I am older myself with the benefit of hindsight, I appreciate even more what they did for us as immigrants in a strange land. I love how hard they worked to assimilate into American culture—their hours at the local high school learning English. It must have been overwhelming and scary for them as we entered school. All the unknowns, language barriers, and cultural differences. I am amazed at how my Dad started and ran a successful business without even knowing how to write in English very well and without a business degree from a university. I love how my Mom supported him and took care of us and our home. The fact that they sent all three of their kids to private colleges is a testament to their capability, determination, and commitment to us kids.

When I think back over my childhood and recall the many days spent at the church they helped build with their friends, I know they were not only driven by their personalities and talents but inspired by God. Who can do what they did without divine intervention and revelation? Before my parents started having children, they, along with a group of their Norwegian friends from the church they attended in Brooklyn, New York, decided that God wanted them to build a church out on Long Island where they were all moving. So, through prayer and hard work, they did. We attended that church throughout my entire childhood, and I grew up surrounded by people who believed in God, served him well, and knew me from the day I was born. That kind of environment affects you deeply. The number of memories I have involving my time at that little church are more than I can say. They're endless and they're good—from the incredible people who taught my Sunday school classes, to the choir director who gave me a musical outlet, and to the friends I sat in the pews with while playing "hangman" or "tic-tac-toe" during a lengthy sermon. I grew up there, got married there, and then dedicated all four of my babies to the Lord, standing in front of that congregation with Mike. Who gets that kind of longevity at a church in this day and age? I'm glad for it and glad that my parents were the kind of people who would build a church and raise their family in the Christian faith. So glad.

But in the midst of all the goodness, there was this brokenness in each one of them that kept me from being able to deal with my pain or even acknowledge it. I am not blaming them for anything. There is no blame. After years and years of wondering why in the world I didn't talk about my pain and deal with it more directly, I have to conclude that I couldn't. I didn't know how or even that I should. A kid needs her parents to help her with the complexities of life, and my parents couldn't help me in this area. If they could have, they would have—that I know.

So, throughout my childhood, my pain went unrecognized by my parents and my pediatrician. The pediatrician never validated my pain and only reinforced the notion that my pain was commonplace, not requiring any special action. When I finally stopped growing at five feet, eight inches, Dr. Broden declared that my ongoing headaches were now being caused by hormones. I couldn't catch a break. So, although frustrated, I was resigned to the facts and continued to accept the reality of pain. Looking back, it makes perfect sense that I never named it, rarely talked about it, and didn't seek help until much later.

During a conversation I had as a teenager with my boyfriend (now husband) regarding the whole "headache thing," I stated how I hadn't grown in a couple of years and was surprised that the headaches hadn't stopped. We were at the high school on a spring afternoon and had just finished a run. Standing by the football stands, the warm sunlight bounced off the aluminum bleachers, and his tanned face and hazel eyes watched me as I nonchalantly asked him how he dealt with *his* headaches.

I waited for his answer as I bent over to stretch my legs. But when I looked up, his eyebrows rose. He shrugged his gorgeous shoulders, "I've never had one," he said.

I stared, and finally whispered, "Never?"

"No, never. I have no clue what a headache feels like," he replied, wiping the sweat off his forehead, still breathing heavily.

I kept after him.

"I'm sure at some point in your life you must've had an ache inside your head! How is it that you've never had a headache?"

My agitation started to take shape as I redid my sweaty, blonde ponytail. How could it be that he never had a headache? Who has *never* had a headache? To think that there were folks who didn't know what a headache felt like made me want to take a swing at him.

I didn't, but knowing he was obviously void of any good advice for me and my head, it was time to go. He dropped me off at home not knowing why the afternoon ended so abruptly. I was mad and needed to digest the fact that not everyone had headaches.

I laid on my bed, door shut, mulling over this new discovery. How did I miss this? It was as if I were born blind, not knowing that others could see. It was *that* surprising. I had always taken comfort assuming we were all in pain together. I believed pain came in varying degrees and frequencies, but I never imagined that some people were headache-free. Other folks had only a few headaches a year? I would never have thought to ask someone how many headaches they had per year. I assumed people's headaches varied per month or week, in severity and duration, but never imagined that there were those who had just a few here and there—or none at all.

Two thoughts stuck with me following that conversation. First, I was confronted with the fact that there really was something wrong with me. Second, I knew I had no interest in finding out what it was. What if there was a simple solution to this lifelong problem? What a fool I would be. All these years of suffering and enduring pain unnecessarily. My mind raced with all the painful days that didn't have to be.

Or, what if the news was grim? What if I had a slow growing brain tumor that had been festering? It definitely would be too late for me, having ignored the signs for so long. I figured I may as well enjoy my remaining time on earth as best I could without a "brain tumor" diagnosis. I know my line of reasoning sounds ridiculous, but I was young.

I also considered the possibility of no answer, good or bad. What if it was complicated and mysterious, sending me to a variety of doctors I didn't like or trust? What if I was born to be a "person with headaches?" What if? I let this new reality sink in over time and adjusted to the fact that, apparently, I was special. For whatever reason, my body manufactured migraines like Ford did cars. When I finally realized that most folks didn't push through this kind of pain every week, it also made me feel lonely, and I had to fight the jealousy I had towards "the headache-less," reminding myself it wasn't their fault they were un-afflicted.

Realizing not everyone battled headaches, I decided that I would continue to endure them in silence. I had the example of my mom whom I admired. I watched her quietly endure life, and it seemed a dignified, reasonable way to go. Anyway, I wanted to be known for my goodness, not my pain. Who wants to be known for their pain? I would keep it a secret for sure.

I also found if I mentioned I had a migraine, people altered plans to accommodate me and my annoying head. They would lower the music, calm the laughing, and put away the chocolate and caffeine. So, fearing my friends might turn the volume down for my sake, I decided it was definitely best to keep silent.

Lastly, I chose the silent route because headaches are not cancer. There are people out there with serious illnesses who deserve our sympathy, help, and time. For Pete's sake, I just have headaches. Despite my chronic pain, I have a healthy body that can do just about anything—aside from a split or cartwheel. So, in the face of people with devastating loss and serious illness, I usually found it ridiculous to talk about my headaches, no matter how painful they were.

I learned there were special medications I could take, but initially opted not to. I discovered that a few people I knew took pain medicine, and they seemed, well, unhealthy and addicted. I also had family members who suffered from alcoholism, and I was afraid my genetics could jeopardize any chance of living an addiction-free life if I started with prescription drugs. I figured I had gotten this far without it, why take a chance on medicine that could end up adding to my problem, even if it did dull my pain? I was an expert in dealing with it and quite used to suffering, ignoring, overcoming, pretending, denying, and pushing through—with the help of over-the-counter pills—which sometimes worked and sometimes didn't. I never knew anything different, so it wasn't a big deal to just carry on.

I was seventeen years old when I discovered not everyone suffered migraines like I did. I also realized my pediatrician had been wrong not to take a closer look at my annual complaint. I ended that year with a heavy sigh and a disdain for doctors, and I resigned myself to the fact that my headaches were here to stay. I was what they called "a migraine sufferer," like scores of others.

But God led the people around by the way of the wilderness toward the Red Sea.

Exodus 13:18a, ESV

3

A Long Time Coming

Do not abandon what You have begun in me, but go on to perfect all that remains unfinished.

—Augustine of Hippo[5]

I WENT OFF TO COLLEGE, then graduate school, keeping my pain at bay. He was my secret enemy, and I kept him under wraps. As years went by, the ebb and flow of my headaches continued with varying intensity. Some years were better than others. The tough ones were ridiculously littered with the dastardly things. But no matter how chronic, I was always determined to keep my life about life, not this constant companion. Maybe it was a lifetime of practice, youth, strength, sheer determination, stupidity, skillful denial, God's grace, or all of the above that kept me from fully registering the pain. However accomplished, I am grateful for years of good memories and not just a chronicle of pain and its consequences.

More than anything, I knew my pain could be more than it was. Even though my headaches and migraines were obstacles in my day, they rarely kept me pinned to my bed. I was glad I could carry on despite their company. I saw others around me who suffered far worse circumstances, so I was often thankful for the level of my pain—grateful it wasn't more. Perspective makes a difference, doesn't it? I also knew I hated the pain too much to let it win the battle for my days and this war on my life. But, eventually, it started winning a few. I suppose it was inevitable. Who can sustain this fight?

In 1988, I graduated with my master's in higher education and got a job at a university on Long Island as a director of residential life. I married my high school sweetheart, Michael, who knew me then and knows me now, and we moved into staff housing on campus, which was perfect since Mike was in law school there. I loved working with college kids and living on campus with my new husband, but when you share a home with someone, it's harder to get away with ignoring your problems. Within our first few months of marriage, he urged me to go to a doctor about my migraines. He couldn't ignore my pain as easily as I could. So, I did.

I found a good doctor through my colleagues at the university and paid her a visit. She recommended a brand new preventative migraine medicine that I would have to take every day whether I had a migraine or not. The thought of taking a drug every day overwhelmed me for multiple reasons, so I turned it down. I was afraid of using a new drug and exposing myself to possible (unknown) side effects. Daily medication seemed too risky. Regardless, I liked my new doctor. She was kind, and, with my rejection of a daily preventative drug, she recommended a pain killer I could take when a migraine was brewing. I reluctantly acquiesced. My younger brother was a recovering alcoholic, and it was enough to watch him suffer and make his way out of that pit. I worried about my own DNA with respect to addiction. Would these pain killers turn into something I couldn't control? My brother wasn't the only one in our family who struggled with this illness. But, I needed something, and a strong pain killer was a welcome addition to my coping arsenal.

Those early years of marriage were filled with law school, new jobs, plus the fun of being young and in love. Mike and I had dated on and off since high school, mastering the art of "the long-distance relationship." During our first years of marriage, I couldn't get over the fun and comfort of finally living in the same place and being together day after day. We were 24 years old when we got married and, in many ways, still kids. We both had a lot of growing up to do, and it was fun to do it together. We figured out our careers, dreamed about the life we wanted to create, thought about the possibility of our own children, places we wanted to go, where we might want to settle down, who we wanted to be, and dialogued about where our faith fit into it all. As with most, our twenties were a great time of personal growth and self-actualization.

My personal faith was still alive and well. Often when a child leaves home, their family's faith is abandoned. You just never know if the faith kids grow up with will continue to be relevant or desirable once they start lives of their own. I remember leaving for college and waking up that first Sunday in my college dorm, realizing I didn't have to go to church anymore if I didn't want to. I was on my own. This was my life now and I could make my own choices about how I spent my time and where I spent it. It felt glorious. I rolled over and went back to sleep, wondering if my faith would survive this new freedom.

But, it did. My relationship with God was deep and wide from my years with him growing up. I continued with church, Bible study and worship during college, and when Mike and I got married, it was something we shared, enjoyed, and counted on. Even in the good times, I found life needed a greater power—a greater companion. Because God is infinitely more than I can imagine, pursuing my faith was incredibly satisfying as he proved himself over and over again to be the million things I needed and desired. I found my relationship with God getting more personal during my twenties, and my faith continued to grow.

As far as I had come in my journey with God, I still believed that he could only help me with my migraines if he healed me. In my mind, there was no other option. I loved having conversations with God about anything and everything, but for some reason when it came to my migraines, my prayers were limited to a cry of headache obliteration and healing. I never thought to ask him for strength, perseverance or whatever else may have been helpful. I would constantly revisit my request for healing, but when the answer was another "no," the conversation ended. "Healer" was the only role I thought he could possibly play in all of it. If he didn't heal me, we didn't have much to talk about when it came to my pain. I don't know why I thought God was limited to that singular task when it came to me and my migraines. I considered myself on my own with the rest of it.

In my late twenties, the pain was starting to wear me down and it began to elbow its way out from my deep places. Sharing life with Mike prevented me from living in denial, and I just didn't have the strength or reserve to override the pain anymore. My will and capacity to hold it at bay were all used up, and I was scared. If I fully succumbed to pain's presence, would it dominate my life? By openly admitting I suffered, would it dictate my days or define my personality? Lead me to bathe in self-pity? I wasn't sure.

Before I could give the pain too much attention, another issue surfaced. Mike and I moved to Philadelphia after he finished law school. We were 26 years old. Mike accepted a job at a firm in Center City, and I started an event planning business. We were busy with our careers, enjoying life in the heart of Philadelphia, and still reveling in the fact that we were married when one day I bragged to Mike that I never got my period. I had just been out with some friends who were moaning about theirs, and the thought was fresh in my mind. I had irregular periods which I attributed to my leanness and involvement in athletics through high school and college, but now I never got them at all. I didn't want to get pregnant, so it didn't present itself as an issue to me, only a bonus—until I saw Mike's face.

"Never?" he said, looking concerned.

"Yup, never," I responded with a smile.

"Eileen, don't you think you should see a doctor? It can't be good that a woman your age doesn't get her period. That is not normal and probably not healthy." He looked serious and had a good point.

I can be a bit clueless sometimes, but when a voice of reason speaks, my ears perk up. Of course, he was right. I made an appointment with a doctor immediately, and we began the process of figuring out why in the world I wasn't working right. It didn't take them long to figure out I had a bad case of endometriosis and what had seemed like a stroke of luck was now just bad news. The absence of a period is *not* a good thing for a woman in her twenties. Up until that point in my life, I hadn't thought much about having a family of my own. The hard fact that I didn't ovulate and may not be able to get pregnant crystallized my thoughts on the subject, though. I wanted kids, and I wanted to birth them myself … badly. I was 27 years old, and all of a sudden it felt like I was running out of time on a dream I didn't even realize I had.

Without much delay, my surgery was scheduled. The doctor's plan was to go in and tear away the fibers from the endometriosis and free my reproductive system so that it could function properly again. At least that was how I understood it. My fallopian tubes were being strangled by fibers and there wasn't an egg small enough to squeeze through and make the trip through the mess to my uterus and grow into a baby. The surgery wasn't a promised solution, but it was definitely needed and a place to start. I had my pre-op meeting and blood work done in preparation for the following week's procedure. It's funny how a seemingly benign conversation with Mike one evening had turned into this mess. I was glad to know what was going on and ready to try and solve it with the hope of one day being able to get pregnant, but it was at this appointment that my doctor advised me to keep my hopes in check and prepare for the likelihood that *I would not be able to get pregnant.* Shocking to hear.

I walked out of the doctor's office at the fertility clinic trying to digest her completely unsettling statement. I wasn't prepared for it, and my heart sank. A wave of grief started to roll in. I called Mike as soon as I got back to our apartment. He was at work and thankfully picked up the phone. I could barely get the words out, but as soon as I did, he made the quick four block walk to our apartment. I cried alone until he got there. Once home, we prayed through our tears for God to make a way and give this bad news a happy ending.

There's a type of crying that only comes with grief. It's exhausting, messy, and cleansing all at once. Releasing all that emotion as we pleaded with God brought me to a point of surrender. This was out of my hands. I would do all I could do, but God was going to have to save me from despair. Mike and I pulled ourselves together and got ready to go out for dinner. All that crying made me hungry. As we left our apartment, I could feel God's peace, and I believed God had heard our cry for help. I had no idea how he would save me from all this, but it felt like he already had.

The weekend before my surgery I promised my brother Kevin I'd come up to New York to celebrate his one-year sobriety anniversary. College life had sucked him into a deep dark hole, and he drank himself silly in the name of fun. I was so proud of the progress he had made in the past year—figuring out the "why's" of his drinking and how to break free. I jumped on the New York bound express train so he could feel my support and love firsthand. I remember sitting on that train, staring at the endometriosis brochures from the doctor's office, trying to resolve the worst-case scenario. I imagined not being able to have children and all I wouldn't get to experience. I thought about babies, toddlers, teenagers and weddings I'd never get to plan. I imagined the graduations we would never attend and family pictures we'd never take. I decided right then and there that if I couldn't get pregnant, I would adopt. Somehow, I would be a mother, and if it wasn't for my own biological children, it would be for someone else's. There was no way I wouldn't experience parenthood and have other human beings to unleash my love on. No possible way. So, adoption it was. My surprisingly quick decision put my mind and my heart at rest. I was going to be a mother, and I was excited. The train arrived at Penn Station, and I made the transfer to the Long Island Railroad feeling better.

Back in Philly, Mike mulled over the conversation I had with the doctor at that last appointment. It upset him that the doctor would tell me such discouraging news when I was there alone. Mike was also obviously struggling with the possibility of us not being able to get pregnant. He always looked forward to being a dad one day and had his own emotions to work through while I was away. He couldn't let go of the fact that the doctor had told me the news without him being there, and he decided he wanted to address it with her. So, unbeknownst to me, Mike called the doctor's office to offer some friendly advice for the benefit of future patients or, more likely, just to give her a piece of his mind. The doctor ended up returning his call, listened courteously for a bit, and, when things started to get heated, abruptly interrupted to ask if she could go over the results she had just received from my pre-op blood tests. His heart sank and he sat down to hear the news. Could the news be even worse?

Life is unpredictable, isn't it? It can change on a dime. You never see it coming until it's upon you. It was a crazy weekend on many levels. Here I was celebrating my 25-year-old brother's sobriety. How in the world did he get himself into such a mess? Of course, I was thrilled about his rehab success, but I was also simultaneously heartbroken that my twenty-something year old brother had felt the need to numb himself by getting drunk. If only he could've processed his pain in a healthy way, he would have avoided this addiction that caused so much trouble and additional pain. It was incredibly sad.

My brother's struggle with addiction and my endometriosis brought a new perspective. My pursuit for migraine relief was, for the moment, on the back burner. Funny how your circumstances recalibrate your life. Who has time for migraine relief when your brother is fighting for his life and you're considering the possibility of not being able to have your own children? I hoped to pick up my pursuit down the road, just not now.

I tried to focus on the positive—which there was plenty of. Kevin was successful with the rehab program and seemed committed to an alcohol-free life. He was processing the issues that had led him to drink and finding his strength in a loving God and family who adored him. Honestly, you don't get much better than my brother. When it comes to kindness, gentleness, and loyalty, he is it. No one could want a happy life for him more than me. He was going to be okay, and it could've been a terrible ending. He could've killed himself in a car wreck or something, but he didn't. He was here and life was getting better for him. I was so thankful. We all were.

I was also thankful that I had a plan forward. My recent news had an answer. If I couldn't get pregnant, there was a baby out there somewhere needing Mike and me. I didn't know how we would find each other, but we would.

We had a little celebration for Kevin at my parent's house over dinner, and before dessert was ready, the phone rang. It was Mike. I was sure he was calling to congratulate Kevin, and everyone in the room yelled out their "hello's." He was quiet and told me I had better sit down. He had spoken to my doctors and had news.

My heart raced as I lowered myself into the chair. My family stared at me, sensing something was wrong.

"What's the matter?" I asked Mike as I clutched the receiver.

"Well, I called the doctor to ream her out about delivering such painful news without me there, and she shared the results from your blood test," he said.

The thought of ovarian cancer crossed my mind, and I held my breath as he continued.

"Eileen, they don't know how it is even possible, but you are pregnant," he finished.

I was speechless. In shock. My brain was trying to register this incredible, unexpected news. My mom, dad, brother and sister were staring at me, and I eventually shouted out, "I'm pregnant!" My parents and siblings celebrated as I tried to get the details out of Mike and relay them to my family gathered around me. How in the world could this be? What did the doctor say? Are you sure? How far along?

Mike and I talked for a while, ecstatic over the great news. It was a miracle and we were overwhelmed by God's grace to us. It felt like we just won lotto. The long infertility road ahead of me had been dramatically cut short. Now, instead of surgery, doctor visits, adoption research and who knows what else, I was free to enjoy good news, eat well and plan for our first child to arrive. Can you imagine how happy we were? My brother's sobriety anniversary festivities turned into a double celebration. It looked like God was redeeming our dire circumstances and making all things good. We were so thankful and elated. I couldn't wait to get back on the train to Philadelphia and go celebrate with Mike. We were going to be parents. Absolutely brilliant news.

At our follow-up doctor appointments, the staff shared their shock and surprise regarding my pregnancy. They didn't say it was a miracle, but I believe they secretly thought it was. I could see it in their eyes and smiles. They counseled us about how a pregnancy is the best therapy for endometriosis and if we were wanting more than one child, we should just keep going. The longer we waited in between pregnancies, the more time the endometriosis had to grow back and cause major reproductive issues again. We knew we wanted to have more than one child, so we registered their advice and would follow it.

My pregnancy was healthy and normal. I ate like crazy and gained an enormous amount of weight while reveling in the fact that I was with child. The migraines were consistent, and I tried to avoid all medicines despite the pain. The day of our first son's birth was spent in Rittenhouse Square near our apartment in Philadelphia. I was committed to doing most of my labor outside of the hospital. A natural approach. Mike and I walked and talked. I remember drinking fresh lemonade throughout the day and then finally, when unable to bear the pain, heading for Pennsylvania Hospital. My water had already broken, and I had trouble getting from the parking garage inside the building. It was June 27, 1992. I still remember holding onto the warm bricks on the outside of the hospital just trying to make it to the entrance. Brutal. I questioned my natural approach, wishing I was in a hospital bed anesthetized. I won't bore you with the details, but soon thereafter our son was born. He was gorgeous, healthy and nine-pounds-six-ounces big.

What was interesting at his birth was his naming. We of course had a list of boy's and girl's names at the ready. We didn't know the sex of our baby until his birth, so we were ready with both lists. Holding him in the hospital, Mike and I couldn't land on a name from the list. None of them seemed right. I remember looking at Mike and saying, "I think his name is Matthew." We didn't have that name on our list, but Mike agreed without hesitation. We wanted our first son to have Mike's name, so it was Matthew Michael Sommi. Later that day, Mike and I talked about how funny it was that his name wasn't on our list and how clear it was to both of us that his name was to be Matthew. I asked Mike to look up the name's meaning in our "baby name book" hoping "Matthew" meant something good. Mike sat on the edge of my hospital bed and flipped through the little book. He smiled as he spoke and told me "Matthew" was a Hebrew name meaning "gift of God." And, there you have it—Matthew, our gift from God.

Mike and I moved back to Long Island from Philadelphia in 1992, soon after Matt was born. Mike decided to join my dad at his construction company and take a break from his law career. We rented an apartment overlooking Northport Harbor—a perfect spot for a young family. Matt and I would spend our days at the park, strolling through town and watching the boaters and fishermen come and go from the town dock. I loved being a mom and couldn't think of a better, more fulfilling responsibility. So, when Mike and I realized I needed to go back to work if we were going to buy a home of our own sooner rather than later, I was crushed. Matt was 12 months old and I couldn't imagine not being with him every second of the day, but Long Island was an expensive place to live, and we needed my income to be able to save enough for a down payment. I called my colleagues at the university and interviewed for the assistant director of residential life position and got the job. Mike, Matt, and I moved back on campus. We knew we would be able to save quickly with staff housing and the extra income. We all settled into life on campus nicely. Matt's daycare center was on campus near my office; Mike had full use of the recreation center again; I loved my job, and we were thankful for it all.

While Mike was working at my father's construction company, an opportunity arose in New York City with the firm he worked for in Philadelphia. They had a small New York office and were looking for a lawyer to come in and manage it. This was a great opportunity for him, and, even though he was enjoying the construction business, he decided to return to the firm. There were a lot of changes in our first years of marriage. It's good to be young and nimble on your feet.

During this time, I became pregnant again. We were following the doctor's advice to have our children close together to continue combatting the endometriosis. After finishing up work one day and walking over to the daycare center to pick up Matt, a strong wave of nausea hit me. I vomited into a nearby garbage can while students walked by. Hard to look professional at that moment, but I was too sick to care. One of my student staff members graciously came close and asked in a whisper if I had a long night. I knew she was joking, but I couldn't think of laughing. She handed me a napkin and walked with me through campus to the daycare center. Like I said, I really loved working with college students.

Our second son, Cole Thomas, was born in 1994 while at Hofstra University. We were so thrilled to have another healthy son, and Matt couldn't have been a happier or prouder big brother. Soon after Cole was born, I let the university know I would be leaving. We had saved enough for a down payment on a small house, and I was ready to be home with my boys, though sad about leaving my career and the extra income. Life often requires meaningful sacrifices. I knew it would be worth it.

We were grateful to be able to have one of us home with the kids. It is not easy to be home full-time raising those babies, but it is rewarding and wonderful. Our new house was in a small neighborhood in one of Long Island's charming north shore villages and was filled with young families. Those days unfolded out of our homes, into our yards and down the sidewalks with the other neighborhood kids. We let them run, play, ride their tricycles and enjoy the simplicity of being kids. We read hundreds of story books, took countless walks around the block, made mud pies, played with turtles, turned our living room into tent villages, baked, danced, and enjoyed the plastic castle and endless stash of Legos crammed in our basement all while waiting for Mike to get home from New York City each night. When his car turned the corner, he was welcomed home by all the neighborhood kids, including ours, running alongside his car screaming with delight. Mike would confess that those homecomings are some of his best memories from those years. A hero's welcome each day—and much deserved. What a great way to end a long day at work.

We had our beautiful daughter Katherine Ingrid while living there. The thought of having a girl was something I couldn't even contemplate. Even though I longed for a daughter, I just assumed I was someone who made boys after having two of them. When she was born and Mike announced we had a baby girl, I couldn't have felt more blessed. Boys and a girl! Mike and I couldn't have been happier that night as we held baby Katherine. I will never forget it. When we drove home from the hospital, I remember seeing all the pink balloons floating above our mailbox. Mike's dear parents were there with Matt and Cole, and they all ran out to welcome us home. It was such a happy scene, and my heart was overflowing being surrounded by such love and blessing.

One of the benefits of motherhood was the new reality of only having a couple migraines a month. Even when I got one, the severity and duration was less than normal. Maybe having children would bring an end to the pain. I hoped they would continue to lessen and I would remain in this manageable state.

Although our family felt full, Mike and I still felt like someone was missing. Having our babies back-to-back was working to ward off the endometriosis, and there was no issue getting pregnant, thankfully. When Katherine was almost one, I believed I was pregnant yet again. I took a pregnancy test when Mike was at work, and it was negative. I was surprised, but relieved because the three were still so little and needed a lot of time and attention. I figured it was a good thing.

Soon after I took that test, I began experiencing acute abdominal pain. I thought it was my period starting up again and the bad cramping was from the endometriosis moving back in, somehow causing everything to hurt more than normal. Throughout the day, the pain continued. I asked my neighbor Trish if she had anything stronger than Tylenol, and she did. I took her pain killers, and it helped a bit. As the evening started, the pain began to build. Mike had finally arrived home, and we got the kids to bed early. I couldn't get comfortable and was beginning to think this was more than bad cramping. I have had bad pain with my period because of endometriosis, but this was different.

There is a moment when you are dealing with pain and it turns a corner. In one moment, you're suffering through it—persevering— and in the next, the instant when the pain moves up the scale, you know it's bigger than you. If you've ever swam in the ocean, it's when you know you are literally in over your head. The waves are too big, the undertow too strong, your body too weak, and you're in big trouble. By late that night, I knew I was in over my head. It was more than I could handle. I couldn't even muster up a prayer for help but hoped God had a plan. I screamed to Mike to get me to a hospital. My insides felt like they were being ripped apart, and for the first time in my life, I thought I might die. Mike frantically called our neighbor to ask him to stay with the kids while he took me to the hospital. Ross ran right over; they carried me to our car, and Mike sped off, racing to the emergency room while I cried and panicked in the back seat, wondering what in the world was happening.

During the car ride, my pain level started to go down. We got ourselves to the emergency room and the doctor on call did some blood work. I laid there while Mike rubbed my back. It felt good to be in relief. I was so tired and still wondering what had exploded inside of me. That's what it felt like. An internal explosion.

The doctor returned to our room and declared, "Congratulations! You are pregnant!"

Mike stopped rubbing my back, and I peered at the doctor through my hair that was covering my face. What was wrong with this guy? Couldn't he see the state I was in? Why was he smiling? He honestly looked as if he was ready to pop a bottle of champagne. There was such a disconnect. Obviously, if I was pregnant, there was something terribly wrong. He then told us we could pull ourselves together and head back home when we were ready. On his way out the door, he said, "Congratulations again!"

It was the twilight zone.

Dazed and confused, we gathered our things and slowly headed toward the exit. Right before we reached the door, I heard the nurse at the front desk call out to us. We turned to look at her. She was young, and I could tell it took a lot for her to speak up.

"I don't think you should leave," she said, staring right into my eyes.

"Why, what do you think is the matter?" I was searching her face for an answer. I knew she knew something.

"I think you may have an ectopic pregnancy, and it would be dangerous if you left. Don't leave." she bravely counseled.

I could sense it was a big deal for her to override the doctor's orders. I immediately knew she was right. It made sense.

"The doctor on call is about to change shifts and I think the next doctor will be more helpful. Stay and let him see you," she finished.

Mike and I turned around, and the nurse got a bed ready for us. I could feel the pain starting again and got scared. The new doctor had just arrived, and the nurse updated him. I told him I was afraid the pain was coming back and begged for an IV drip of morphine or something so I wouldn't have to feel it again. He hooked me up. I don't really remember all the details of what happened. Mike talked to the doctor for a few minutes and before I could even digest what was happening the doctor and nursing team were running me and my gurney down the hall towards the operating room. The doctor quickly told me they had to operate immediately. He explained that I was experiencing an ectopic pregnancy and they needed to rush and catch it before it burst my fallopian tube which could result in extensive internal bleeding. I suppose the pain meds were taking hold of me because I was not phased and thought they could do whatever they wanted to do as long as I didn't have to feel that pain again. I was asleep before we got to the operating room.

The good doctor completed the surgery and removed my fallopian tube and when I woke up, he and Mike were by my bedside. He told me I must have angels watching over me. He explained, "Eileen, your pregnancy had already burst your fallopian tube, and when this happens, you run the risk of dying from extensive internal bleeding. But, somehow, the membrane from the tube got caught and kept all the bleeding contained like a rubber barrier in an ocean oil spill. It saved your life."

I remember thinking I was going to die when Mike and our dear neighbor loaded me into the car rushing me to the hospital. I am sure it must have burst long before we even got to the hospital. How that little membrane contained the bleeding while I was being moved around is beyond me. A miracle. It wasn't my day to die, but, unfortunately, my baby didn't make it. Straight to the arms of Jesus her soul must've flown. I had a strong feeling the baby was a girl. I sure hope to meet her in heaven one day.

Before leaving the hospital, I asked my dear doctor if I would be able to get pregnant again. He told me I still had one fallopian tube left, so yes. I left Huntington Hospital grateful and full of hope despite the sadness over our loss. Not soon after, I was pregnant with Grace Eileen.

I was pregnant six times between the ages of 28 and 35. We gave birth to four beautiful children: Matthew Michael, Cole Thomas, Katherine Ingrid, and Grace Eileen. I had one miscarriage in between Matthew and Cole and the ectopic pregnancy between Katherine and Grace. We followed the doctor's advice, and my endometriosis was kept at bay, allowing my body to function well. I know many women who have found themselves at the fertility clinic and never able to get pregnant. Why we were able and so many are not is beyond my understanding. I just know I am thankful for what happened to us. Being a mom has been my greatest joy and privilege. Having my own biological children is a gift beyond measure. I also know that if God didn't allow it, he would have allowed something else that would have been equally beautiful.

My "childbearing years" were good years, and I was getting used to my migraines being less frequent and severe. One of my migraine triggers is definitely hormones. I was grateful because I honestly don't know how I could've managed it all without the relief. It was reason enough to keep having children.

Pain relief was just one of the many blessings of those years. We knew the grace we were experiencing was a gift from God. Our children. Our marriage. Our home. Our church. Our neighbors. All of it. Amidst the sleepless nights, terrible two tantrums, scraped knees, and crocodile tears, there was so much goodness. We read the ancient stories to the kids and taught them the greatness of God's ways—the beauty of kindness, forgiveness, and love—as best we could. Even though it was stressful getting everyone ready for church on Sunday morning, it was always worth being there for the friends, teaching, and singing—a great place to start the week and be reminded of who we are and who God is.

When Grace was just 5 months old, I thought I was pregnant again. I was driving somewhere and had the urge to stop at our local deli for a bag of potato chips and lemonade—a craving that only arose when I was pregnant. I panicked and called Mike to pick up a pregnancy test on his way home from work. Once the kids were in bed that night, we met in the bathroom. I peed on that stick and gave it to Mike. While we waited for the results, I had a meltdown. I was tapped out with four kids and the thought of adding another person to the mix tipped my scales. Mike reassured me that we would get the help I needed. We would figure it out and make it work. He talked while I cried. The pregnancy test was negative, and I exhaled. It was clear we needed to be done having children. Mike made an appointment with his old college buddy who was a urologist. Dr. Wagner would make sure Grace would always be our fourth and final. As tempting as it is to keep having babies—because they are beyond words—everyone has their threshold and four was mine.

Seven years of major migraine relief made me think I was probably beyond the chronic pain at this point. But, once Grace finished nursing, they returned with force and regularity. I couldn't believe they were back. Having had relief made it feel even worse. The relief objectified my pain, and I wasn't tolerant anymore. I couldn't accept it. Grace was a few months old when it all came crashing in on me.

Before Grace was born, we had moved from Northport to Cold Spring Harbor. We bought a historic home that needed a lot of work. Our new old house was a mess when we got it with an odor strong enough to kill a rabbit. Being pregnant with Grace during the renovation made me even more sensitive to the odor since, for some reason, my sense of smell was always heightened when pregnant. It was nauseating. I remember showing the house to my dad, the builder. As a professional, he understood the location and the value of the property, but the house eluded him. He knew we would need his expertise and help to restore it and honestly believed it wasn't worth it. However, he couldn't resist my enthusiasm over the potential of it all and eventually joined us in figuring out a solution. I also had the help and vision of my brother who worked with my father as an architectural designer. How lucky were we to have our family so perfectly suited to help us with a project this overwhelming.

There was a lot of dust, bricks, painting, demolition, and work crews mixed in with my three young kids and a baby girl that first year. It was a mother's nightmare and a kid's paradise, complete with piles of dirt, bulldozers in the yard, and a constant parade of interesting people to interact with from the electrician to the carpenters. Matt, Cole, and Kit thought they had died and gone to heaven. Baby Grace was oblivious to the chaos and spent those months strapped to my body as I tried to keep her siblings out of danger. In the evenings after the kids went to sleep, Mike and I did what we could to speed up the restoration process until the house was one day not only habitable but inviting.

Those days were intense. I was a young mom with four children in a new neighborhood where I didn't know a soul. Mike had to commute to Manhattan every day for work, which added hours to an already long workday, and I spent most of my time at home trying to contend with the construction and figure out how to cook dinner without a kitchen. It was stressful. My head hurt. I was sleep deprived and washing the dishes in a bathtub upstairs. It wasn't good.

One night while standing outside grilling hotdogs in the side yard with grass up to my knees, I remember thinking it was all too much. My tears started falling onto the grill as my shoulders shook uncontrollably. The kids were literally naked in the backyard covered in mud; I had a migraine; I could hear Grace inside crying as she woke up from a nap, and I thought something has got to change. Even though I didn't want to add to my list of things to do, something inside me crystallized, and I determined in my heart to get help. I needed help with the kids and help with my head. I also needed to stop pretending I didn't need help. What was that about? Who doesn't need help, and what is the shame in it? I needed physical help and supernatural help. And, I needed it quickly.

So, before the hot dogs were done cooking, I knew the next day I would be on the phone making calls to friends, doctors, and someone who could come to the house a few hours a week and simply help me. It was a turning point for me out there in the long grass by the grill. I'm not exactly sure what snapped me out of it in that particular moment, but I suppose I finally had enough. The relief during my pregnancy years had given me needed objectivity. I'm sure my husband's prodding to get help broke through my stubbornness and grit. Maybe my kids covered in mud woke me up. It was also my anger toward the pain that propelled me. Or perhaps, I now thought myself worthy of relief. Whatever the reasons, I was ready to fight. My spell of powerlessness and denial was broken, and I stood eager to wage war and finally obliterate the painful intruder inside my head. It was a supernatural moment. I felt like the spirit of God was blowing through me and giving me motivation, vision, grit, and the power of a warrior to go after this thing. I was 36 years old, and it was about time.

For now we see in a mirror dimly, but then face to face. Now I know in part; then I shall know fully, even as I have been fully known.

I Corinthians 13:12, ESV

4

Waging War

It is common sense to take a method and try it. If it fails, admit it frankly and try another. But above all, try something.

—Franklin D. Roosevelt

PAIN HAD COME TO THE FOREFRONT. It was no longer lurking in the shadows. I picked it up, placed it right in front of me, and turned on the light. I couldn't pretend to ignore it another minute, dodge it another day. Finally, we stood eyeball to eyeball. Feeling brave and unstoppable, I felt God prompting me to start with the truth. A quote from the Bible held me captive with its promise—"The truth will set you free."[6] Yes, I would start there. Freedom from the intruder's oppressive presence and relentless banging was what I wanted.

From that day forward, I gave my best effort to embrace truth at every turn and speak it with every word. A new boldness and confidence was growing in me—an ownership of who I was and what was—minus the fear and ambiguity. Covering up my pain was no longer an option. My subconscious impulse to hide it and be quiet was subsiding and just didn't make sense. Answering questions of well-being with a lie would no longer happen. I would finally speak of my pain, bear the consequences, and maybe, reap the reward of the promise: freedom.

I began with friends, people I trusted. Instead of swallowing my complaint of the day, I started sharing it. As I let truth flow out, fearing the listeners' disbelief, impatience, or apathy, I was stunned by their responses.

I ran into a friend who asked the inevitable "Hey, how's it going?" question. Buttressed by my commitment to truth, I explained I had a migraine that was on its fourteenth day and told him I was at the end of my coping skills along with being utterly exhausted. I couldn't conjure up the energy at this point to inject intonation into my reply. I watched his face for a response, but mostly expected a change of subject or kind pat on the shoulder. As I began to wonder at his silence, I saw his eyes fill with compassion and sorrow as he struggled to respond.

Have to say, I didn't expect that.

Another friend told me she was upset that I had never shared my pain with her. She said I denied her the privilege of caring and praying for me. Certainly didn't mean to do *that.* How could I have underestimated a friend's love to think that she would tire of me if I was, well, a bit of a burden at times?

What a great discovery and relief all of this was. It washed over me like a warm shower, and my heart became full and comforted realizing I wasn't alone and friends wanted to walk with me.

And so it went, surprise after surprise, responses to my pain that I never anticipated. As time passed, I felt my wall begin to crumble as I let the light of friendship into my world of headaches—strengthening me for the battle about to begin. Who knew that complaining wasn't necessarily a bad thing?

My decision to fully address my pain problem sent me into the world of doctors, cat scans, waiting rooms, diets, and chart keeping. Having never fully recovered from my distrust and dislike of my pediatrician years ago, the medical world wasn't a place I wanted to visit. But I had no choice.

Since many of my headaches were lodged in my sinus cavity, I decided my first doctor's visit would be to an ear, nose, and throat specialist who would take a picture of my head and analyze it. I was 99.9% sure I would receive my answer here. I made some medical inquiries through my adult years to try and relieve my pain, but I had never had anyone actually look inside my head. I was sure that at first glance they would see some sort of obstruction behind my face. I wondered about a possible tumor or a sinus cavity covered in polyps. I hoped for some physiological explanation.

The doctor took images of my sinus cavity and once his analysis was complete, he happily stated that "everything looked beautiful."

"What do you mean 'everything looks beautiful'?" I said with disappointment.

"I mean everything looks normal and healthy," the doctor replied.

"If you wouldn't mind taking another look—I'm sure there must be something there, something abnormal. Perhaps if you looked a little deeper?" I pleaded.

"The pictures don't lie. There's nothing wrong. This is good news," he said, growing impatient.

I just stared at him as he handed me a two-ounce, green bottle of nasal spray.

"Here, try this. Spritz it in your nostrils a few times a day. I'm sure it'll help," he said and left the room to go see his next patient.

I sat there stunned on the examining table. What a jackass. I was certain he thought I was exaggerating, or he simply didn't have the brain capacity to comprehend the level and longevity of my pain. I had tried to explain it to him with as much detail as I could, but to no avail. After thirty years of headaches, I gathered my belongings and returned home with a green, two-ounce bottle of nasal spray and started spritzing.

The first bottle didn't help. Nor did the next few dozen or so. So, I gave up and looked for another solution.

My next effort was a trip to the allergist. I had not been to one before and never thought I was allergic to anything. But some allergy ridden friends suggested that my sinus pain and migraines could be an allergic reaction. Based on recommendations, I chose a doctor and made my appointment. My minivan rolled into the medical center's parking lot. Hope prevailed and I made my way to her office.

I opened the office door and felt like I stepped into a dream. The room gleamed white and smelled freshly cleaned while the atmosphere was void of anything unpleasant. I heard a light hum and guessed it must be the air filters busy at work. The hypo-allergenic environment made my head feel lighter, and my hope grew. I watched the doctor and her assistants working behind the counter as I checked myself in and couldn't help but notice their pressed, white uniforms—which enhanced my feeling of wellness. Effective marketing, if nothing else.

Not long after my arrival, the receptionist called my name. The doctor stood at the entrance of her office and motioned me in with a friendly smile. She looked clean and polished just like her surroundings and pointed to a chair across her desk. Her white lab coat and perfectly poised brown hair gave her an air of confidence and relaxed me. I sat down, and we began to get acquainted as we spoke of motherhood and busy schedules before delving into my health history. As I summed up the past thirty years of my life, she appeared intrigued—which was encouraging.

She was troubled that I had put up with headaches since I was a young girl and surprised that I had never been to an allergist. I couldn't begin to explain and simply reminded her it was better late than never. She then began to ask about my headaches and their frequency.

"So, when does the sinus pressure or headache begin? Spring? Summer? Fall?"

"Well, it doesn't begin. It's always there," I said.

"Mmm." She jotted some notes.

"Does your head feel worse in certain environments, after eating certain foods, or being around certain animals?" she continued.

"I can feel worse in a certain environment or season, or after eating certain foods, only to feel my best the next time I'm in that same place or eating that same thing. Honestly, I can't find a pattern to my pain," I said.

"Okay then," she said, bending over her clipboard writing some more.

"Well, why don't we just get started? You sound highly allergic to something," the doctor continued. She looked curious as she pushed her glasses back up her nose. Or was it confused?

They escorted me to an examination room for testing. As I watched her and the assistant walk back and forth between various cabinets in the room gathering vials for my testing, I thought it would be tremendous to be highly allergic to some headache producing substance that could be relieved by allergy medicine.

There were three examining tables in the room; two were occupied—one by me and the other by a young girl getting her allergy shots. I looked on and noticed her familiarity with the process—a couple of questions by the doctor, a lift of the sleeve, the quick injection, a hop off the table, and out the door. Off she went with her antidote. I bet she had no idea how lucky she was.

"Jen, start her on low doses. I'm afraid she's highly allergic to something and we wouldn't want her throat closing up on us," the doctor said to the young assistant now standing in front of me. The doctor gave me a friendly wink and left me alone with Jen.

Jen pricked me with the first substance—grass. She then set the timer and followed the doctor to the other side of the room where the white medicine cabinets were located. As they walked away, I knew they couldn't possibly understand how welcomed a strong allergic reaction would be. I wished I'd break out in hives, or my throat would tighten. *Something* to explain my painful head.

I remained hopeful as the young woman smiled at me and continued scraping and pricking my upper arm with other substances. With a prick and a scrape, she would then set the timer and head for the cabinets to gather the next possibility. When she returned, the two of us would stare at my arm for a reaction. Redness. Puffiness. Swelling. Hives. But with each scrape and prick, my arm remained annoyingly smooth and pale.

We revisited this routine over a series of visits. I became well acquainted with Jen's shiny brown hair and pleasant face as she faced me week after week pricking away at my arm. I studied her to pass the time and became impressed with her focus and professional, friendly demeanor—not to mention her well-groomed eyebrows. As each test ended without an allergic reaction, her lovely eyebrows would rise, and she would let out another "huh."

On my sixth visit, my last prick and scrape tested for reactions to dust and pollen. Once the timer sounded, Jen searched my bicep and believed she saw a reaction. Jen called the doctor over as I continued to study my arm. After some discussion, they agreed I was reacting to the dust and pollen. I wanted to tell them my arm was red from all the pricking and scraping, but my desire to be allergic to something made me hold my tongue. So, I took it as good news that I was allergic, and since dust and pollen are basically everywhere, this particular allergy would explain my constant headaches. I got my medicine and went home with the exciting news.

My husband, Mike, didn't think it was as exciting as I. He, always more practical and logical, thought it would be difficult to control my exposure to dust and pollen in our dusty, old house surrounded by hundred-year-old trees that routinely blanketed our yard with a light green film. But his lack of excitement didn't mean he was lacking in his desire to try. So, we decided to do everything in our power to rid our home of dust. The yard was hopeless, and we trusted the medicine would address that problem.

As we began the assault on our home, I went through the list of suggestions the doctor had given me to help eliminate dust. Having a good vacuum cleaner was listed as number three. Being that my current vacuum was only semi-effective, I decided to dispose of it and go shopping. After some research, I purchased the highly acclaimed German model with the "active HEPA filters" designed to filter out 99.7% of particles and microorganisms. This particular vacuum was specifically recommended for allergy sufferers—of whom I was now one. I figured if you really got what you paid for, this machine was going to be a huge help.

Mike had a company revamp our entire heating and cooling system with more HEPA filters, and I started vacuuming not only my rugs, but the curtains. I washed my bed sheets in scalding hot water to kill any of the dreaded dust mites (number one on the doctor's list) and bought all the appropriate dust cover protectors. I purchased face masks to use when I cleaned (as recommended) and hired a housekeeper to help me keep up with my dusty old house (an obvious perk for my condition). We kept our windows permanently shut to keep the filtered air in and the pollinated, dusty air out. I have to say I missed the breezes and the smell of fresh air in my house, but not enough to jeopardize my chances for relief. I faithfully took my medicine, and yet month after month I woke up in my dust free bed feeling like I had just been hit by a Mack truck.

Allergies didn't appear to be the cause of my pain. It was a huge disappointment.

In time I gathered the energy for a new doctor and another possibility; my heart lightened at the thought of opening my windows again. I wouldn't miss wearing the masks, and, well, I had needed a new vacuum anyway. The housekeeper stayed just in case the cleaner environment was helping a little. She needed the work, and I needed the help; plus, after months of bonding over dust mites, face masks, and the occasional cup of coffee, we were friends. But it was unfortunately time to move on to the next doctor.

Through discussions with some dear friends, I was urged to explore the possibility that I may have an overgrowth of yeast in my system called Candida. I had never heard anything about this condition and decided to do some research. Mike and I explored the internet and came up with websites and lots of literature pertaining to this illness.

As I read, I began to believe that this could possibly be my problem. Candida was under the radar of most doctors, and yet many people suffered from it for years as it went undiagnosed. I read many encouraging stories of people who had suffered similar symptoms, only to have them disappear once they brought the Candida under control.

I was connected with a nutritionist who prescribed a diet and course of action to rid my body of this systemic problem. A girlfriend who suffered headaches and a variety of the "Candida symptoms" decided to join me on this one. After our completion of a lengthy questionnaire and initial meetings with the nutritionist, she declared that we both ranked very high on the Candida scale, and there was no doubt in her mind that we were suffering from this condition. She prescribed THE DIET and appropriate supplements. I remember making her promise me that if I followed this regimen, which I could see was going to be grueling, the Candida would be killed and my headaches would subside. She said that if I followed the plan exactly, with no mistakes, it would.

Now, I like a challenge and her tone had "challenge" all over it. I silently promised myself right there and then that I was going to be her star patient with nary a slip up. I suspiciously believed that she probably figured no one could follow this crazy diet, and when it didn't work, she would be able to say, "Well, if you followed it perfectly it would've worked, but ..." My cynicism and distrust of the medical world were growing.

Hundreds of dollars later, we left her office armed with supplements, ready to embark on eight weeks of body cleansing and yeast killing. I was like a warrior going into battle after hearing the greatest pep talk of the century. I had a bag of hope in my hand and a date assigned to my imminent relief from these overbearing headaches. What more could a girl want?

My girlfriend and I went for one last cup of coffee and a blueberry muffin before we started. I was determined to do this thing right, and I did (minus the small piece of pretzel I succumbed to while shopping one evening).

The diet was strictly limited to foods that would not feed the Candida, basically leaving us with very little to eat. It was weeks of protein and vegetables minus some of the really good proteins and a few of my favorite vegetables. I don't know about you, but I love fruit, carbohydrates, dairy products, and sugar (both natural and processed). To say good-bye to those food categories simultaneously was nothing less than excruciating.

I particularly remember a beach outing with some friends on a glorious day. Food was being passed; the barbecue was releasing the most intoxicating aroma, and friends were raising glasses to toast the end of a great summer. My mouth salivated as I looked on with desire, and just when the thought of breaking the diet would enter my pounding head, I remembered the promise: If I stuck to the diet, I would kill the culprit and get relief from all of this. With my starving body in the center of an aromatic smorgasbord of favorite foods, it was an easy decision. I wanted relief and no temptation would prevent me from getting it.

Through almost daily phone calls with my friend, I made it. I had a string of five days without a headache during that diet, but that was it. I continued with a modified version in case my body needed more time, but aside from my body feeling cleansed, the pain persisted. Another promise broken. I walked away fifteen pounds lighter with a deepened friendship with my "diet partner," but that was it.

I continued to manage my pain with my over-the-counter drug collection ranging from Excedrin Migraine to Goody's Aspirin Powders. I currently didn't have a prescription strength pain killer and knew I needed to remedy that sooner rather than later. Even though these products often have little to no effect, the television commercials for them look so promising. The miserable looking woman on the screen with the furrowed brow and tired eyes reminds me of myself. I listen to the narrator describing her pain and believe if I try their pill again, it will work. The commercial always ends with the woman looking so happy, running through a field of daisies. It makes me hopeful, and for the times they do help, I'm grateful.

During this season of assault, I read a book about a doctor from Africa who not only studied western medicine but also non-traditional medicine. I loved his philosophy and thought if I could have him as my doctor, I might find some answers. As I read his biography on the back jacket, I saw he practiced medicine in New York City, about 20 miles from where I lived. Perfect. I picked up the phone and left a message. I made the call early Sunday morning, and by 9:30am on Monday, the doctor/author was ringing my number. What doctor makes phone calls? I was impressed and grabbed his first available appointment.

I anticipated my appointment as if it were Christmas morning. The day finally arrived, and I rode the train into Manhattan. My head was pounding from a migraine, making the ride pretty uncomfortable. Leaving Penn Station, clutching his book against my chest, I wandered through skyscrapers, searching for his office. My hope soared as my stomach turned. I don't know why I get so nervous with each new doctor, but I do. Perhaps it's all the hope mixed with fear of disappointment.

I finally found his posh looking office and climbed the stairs to the waiting room. When I entered, the difference between the busy city sidewalk and the Zen-like atmosphere of the room struck me. I felt better already. The place had a clean, comforting smell of Sweetgrass. The walls were a neutral, calming taupe color, and the décor was minimal. After I checked in, I sat in the lovely waiting room, mentally re-decorating my entire home. Perhaps my headache problem was an aesthetic one that could be solved simply by giving my old, cluttered farmhouse a new, Eastern design that would somehow clear my nasal passages and relax my head into a pain-free state. When my name was called, I quickly archived those thoughts for another time.

At the end of a long hallway, I found him waiting for me in his office. He reached out his hand and welcomed me into his book-covered room filled with souvenirs from far-away places. He was young, trim, and his glasses made him appear thoughtful and smart. I trusted he was. His demeanor was noticeably serene, and I thought he must have spent the entire morning doing advanced yoga. The difference between him and me seemed as vast as the contrast between the city sidewalk and his waiting room. With a notebook in hand, he calmly started asking me questions, and I began to talk faster than an auctioneer.

I was now accustomed to doctors having approximately two minutes to hear my headache story, so when they say "speak," I go as fast as I can to get as much in as possible before their internal beeper goes off and they make their hasty diagnosis. As I rattled on about my headache history, I realized he was not in a rush, and after each of my monologues, he followed up with a few more questions. I took comfort in his head nodding, and I slowed my speech, suddenly free to speak in more detail, offer extra background and information. He seemed to understand. Even better, he seemed to know something.

Thorough like a detective, I could see his brain working to try and put the puzzle together. It was the first time I felt like a doctor was truly hearing me. At most visits, they look right past you, and you never feel a connection, only the rush of the appointment schedule. How can any doctor figure out what is wrong with somebody without taking the time to thoroughly hear their history? I imagine there are many misdiagnoses and frustrated people in pain out there.

At the end of an hour, we had covered so much ground that I thought we could become friends. I liked yoga, we were both obviously interested in the "art of healing," and I would love to hear about life in Africa. Amazing what a little active listening can do for a person.

When I was done recounting my history, he stated (with a confidence and genuineness that I had yet to encounter in a doctor's office), "I believe I can definitely help you."

He could help me? The words stopped time.

I wanted to fall on my face and hug his ankles. I immediately pictured him pouring over the copious notes he had just taken and staying up to the wee hours of the morning, cross referencing his medical encyclopedias, holistic journals, and case studies. I envisioned my husband and I treating him and his wife to a lovely dinner in the city, raising our glasses to toast the long-awaited victory.

Until I heard him speak of needles.

I'm not really sure how long he'd been talking about acupuncture when I decided to pay attention, but he seemed to want to try it immediately. I sobered up and asked him a few questions of my own. He explained the history and process and told me it had helped many people with various problems through the centuries. And it would be just one of a few things he would like to try to help heal me.

He also explained that from listening to my history, it seemed I had a myriad of things going on in my body. He mentioned my digestive system, hormonal system, adrenal system, and a few other systems. "I was complicated," he said (which I'd heard before, just not from a doctor). But he assured me, over time we would figure it all out.

In the meantime, he wanted to start with some acupuncture to help relieve some of my pressure. As I digested what he was offering, I decided that acupuncture sounded interesting. Who knows, what would happen if he relieved all my pressure points and whatever else those needles could do? Although I'd been known to faint when confronted with a needle, I was not going to refuse a possible remedy.

So we traveled down the pleasant smelling hallway into the acupuncture room—me, my headache, and my new doctor. Upon arrival, he asked if I would remove everything but my undergarments and take my place on the table.

As he left the room to give me some privacy, I wished I knew about this part of my appointment. If I did, I may have prepared myself a little better. Perhaps a little moisturizer on my dry, scaly legs. Perhaps I would've worn my new underwear and not my favorite pink bikini bottoms that were definitely showing signs of aging. I would have certainly shaved my prickly legs and armpits. I reminded myself that doctors are professionals, and they don't care about such things. They see our bodies like a car mechanic views a car—an object to be worked on. He re-entered the room and I kept repeating the words "car mechanic, car mechanic, car mechanic ..." until his conversation and demeanor assured me of his absolute professionalism and disregard for my hairy legs and ripped bikini underwear. I began to relax again.

I definitely wasn't prepared for the size of the acupuncture needles. They were not your average push pins but, rather, thin needles long enough to roast a marshmallow. The doctor told me that he would insert the needles throughout my body and try to relieve the pressure. He also told me to relax, which I was already desperately trying to do. I took a deep breath as he started to insert them into my forehead and down to my ankles. The more needles he inserted the faster my breathing became. When he was done, I looked like a porcupine in headlights.

Lying there on the table, almost naked, covered in needles, with twangy, Eastern music playing in the background, I began to freak out.

"What's the matter?" the doctor asked, leaning over to make eye contact through the forest of needles.

What was the matter? Can you imagine? I was barely dressed, alone in a room with a man I met an hour ago, covered in long needles, and he was asking me "What's the matter?"

As tears arrived, my entire being fixated itself on the needles poking out of my skin. I realized the twangy music was putting me over the edge.

"You've got to shut off this stupid music and put on Mozart!" I blurted out. The crazy sensation of making the needles on my face move while talking freaked me out further, and I went from bad to worse.

He hurried out of the room and within seconds remedied the music. He re-entered the room.

"Eileen, please slow down your breathing," he said without being able to hide the worry on his face.

I stared at him in a panic, unable to do it.

"Like this. Copy me." The good doctor started to breathe in and out slowly.

He continued for a while and willed my breathing into a slower rhythm. I knew he wouldn't stop until I joined him—which I eventually did.

As I slowed my breathing, he asked if I was alright. I didn't dare speak again with needles all over my face and mustered up an "uh-huh."

"Good job. You've got to try and relax. Keep your breathing slow and steady," he gently commanded as he placed a small bell in my hand.

"If you need me just ring this bell and I'll come back. Just remember to relax. Deep breath in and slowly exhale." His voice faded as he left the room, shutting the door quietly behind himself.

As I watched him leave, I was sure he was wondering where the sensible woman he had met in his office went. I was disappointed in myself.

Alone, without my new doctor and forced to deal with my breakdown, I was determined to get a grip. There was no help in sight, and none would be coming since I couldn't figure out how to wave that silly bell with needles all over my arm. I let the bell fall to the floor and conjured up some of my Lamaze techniques from my baby birthing days. I started to slow my breathing and calm down. Mozart definitely helped, and I picked a spot on the ceiling to focus on instead of trying to count the needles that were rising and falling with each breath I took.

I stared at the spot on the ceiling and relaxed. As I did, my emotional wall seemed to crash down. I began crying like a baby. Now what? Oblivious to the reason for my tears, I worried what the doctor would think of me and wished for a free hand to blot my wet face. Already embarrassed by my panic attack, did the doctor also have to witness an emotional breakdown? Oh brother.

I decided that I either needed serious counseling for some problem I was totally unaware of, this was truly an overwhelming situation, or acupuncture makes people cry. I would make sure to ask the doctor about it and wept until he returned.

He walked toward the table with a sympathetic grin on his face.

"You did great," he said while removing the needles like candles from a birthday cake.

"You know as well as I that I didn't, but thanks anyway," I replied, reaching for the box of tissues. "I have to ask you if my reaction to the acupuncture was unusual."

"Well, I haven't had anyone panic quite like you, but many people cry," he said with the kind of smile that strengthens a soul.

(Somewhat defensively I didn't get it. A panic attack seemed a natural response to such a strange scenario. I was struck by the fact that there is a patient population who come to his office and are able to remain calm with footlong needles inserted into their bodies. Impressive really.)

While pulling out the last needle from my ankle area, he continued, "As your pressure points are relieved, your body often lets out what it's holding inside and relaxes to the point of a good cry. Make sense?"

"Hmm. I suppose these headaches are making me sadder than I realized," I said with a sigh.

"Speaking of which, how does your head feel? Is the headache gone?"

I reluctantly told him it was alive and well.

He cocked his head sideways, looking surprised with a hint of concern. "I was sure the acupuncture would give you some immediate relief," the good doctor responded. "Well, why don't you dress and meet me in the reception room?"

I was exhausted, and I slipped on my clothing and digested the fact that the acupuncture didn't stop my head from pounding. For all the effort, it would have been nice if it had. Once dressed, I went to the restroom to wash my face. The cold water was renewing, as was having clothes on instead of needles. I inhaled the Sweetgrass smell and went to meet the doctor. Feeling vulnerable after the acupuncture debacle, I could barely look him in the eye.

He gave me supplements and told me to make another appointment. I told him I would need to think about it. On the train ride back home, I realized there was no quick solution on the horizon. No magic pill. I believed this doctor could help me but knew it would be a long, involved process, and his office was just too far away. If I wasn't so busy with the kids at home, he would've been my guy. It made me sad, but what can you do?

After that visit, I took a break from doctors. I was drained, discouraged, and my life was calling me. All this effort was time consuming and self-focused. I had four children who needed me, along with a life, house, and husband wanting some attention. Who has time to be sick? Life is busy and each day full, making it nearly impossible to carve out time for yourself, not to mention entire days sitting in waiting rooms and doctors' offices.

When my energy was replenished and my mindset ready, I made another appointment with a new doctor who had been recommended by a friend. He told me that this doctor helped many people he knew with ailments their regular doctors couldn't cure. I liked the sound of that.

For God gave us a spirit not of fear but of power and love and self-control.

2 Timothy 1:7, ESV

5

The Waiting Room

Our pursuit of God is successful just because He is forever seeking to manifest Himself to us.

—A.W. Tozer[7]

TALK ABOUT DISASTER. My appointment with this new doctor was for 9:00 a.m. I had three kids to get ready and on the school bus at 8:20, and the office was a 45-minute drive from home. My husband, Mike, was driving with me so that he could watch our youngest daughter Grace while I met with the doctor. When the main road leading to the highway was blocked by detour signs, I knew we were in trouble. We found ourselves meandering at a snail's pace through suburban neighborhoods as the clock ticked on.

By the time we reached the highway, we had about 7 minutes to get to the doctor's office – which would be impossible. We moved as fast as we could without killing ourselves or anyone else on the road, and I could feel my stress level rise as the clock moved past my long-awaited appointment time. In the end, we were half an hour late.

Mike dropped me off at the front entrance to the office, and I ran through the empty waiting room up to the glass window and introduced myself to the smiling receptionist.

I explained the unexpected road construction and apologized for being late.

She looked down at her schedule shaking her head.

"Well, I'm so sorry, but we will have to reschedule you for another day."

She stated it so plainly as if it were nothing. My blood boiled immediately.

Now, you have to understand the anticipation that accompanies these doctor visits. The recommendations are always emphatic, and my hope ignites. I daydream about the day I won't have to deal with all these headaches, and I begin to believe this particular doctor will be the one who will unlock the mystery. So, I enter each office with great expectations, which inevitably sets me up for great disappointment. Also, most good doctors have a long waiting list for new patients, and this one was no exception. I had waited four months to get this appointment. And, lastly, I am usually in a lot of pain, still desperate for relief. So when the receptionist told me I was too late and would have to reschedule, I began to unravel.

"I'm sorry, but I've waited months for this appointment, and we're only a half hour late, and your waiting room is completely empty."

"Yes," she said still smiling, "but we are booked today and if I put you in now, the entire day will get backed up. Let's see when the next opening will be. Hmmm. Next month, we have …"

I interrupted her and heard my voice getting louder.

"I cannot wait until next month. My husband took the morning off work for this; I've already waited *four* months, and my head is currently about to explode from pain. I need to see him today." I stared at her with desperate eyes and noticed she was unmoved.

"This is crazy," I continued. "Your waiting room is absolutely empty. Please, I am begging you to let me see the doctor."

Still smiling, she said, "I'm sorry. We're very booked."

Did I just land in hell? I had a couple of choices at that moment. I could either jump over the counter and strangle her or run outside to my husband and tell him to do something. Luckily, I chose the latter. I told him what had happened and pleaded with him to use his skills of persuasion and get me in there. Mike was a lawyer, and I figured his years of trial experience could be put to great use in this moment.

I watched him walk into the building with the resolve of a champion. He would fight for me and win. I could see it in his face and eyes. I leaned against our minivan, begging God to break through and make it happen. After a couple of minutes, Mike came out to the car and said that the best they could do was see me late that afternoon. I lost it.

On this particular day, my migraine marathon was entering week two, which meant I was at the bottom of my survival bag of tricks. My appointment this morning was what I had been clinging to for the last ten days. The afternoon was filled with kids coming home from school, and it would mean that my daughter Grace would have to be with me at the appointment since Mike needed to eventually go to work. It was too complicated and hard (at that moment) to manage. Under normal circumstances, I could have rallied, called friends to watch the kids and made it happen. But I was more burnt out on all of this than I realized.

I started to cry inconsolably and left my husband and little girl at a loss for ways to help. I decided a walk would do me good. I left my bewildered family at the van, and started moving as fast as I could to any place away from there. I was exasperated and mad (mostly at God) that I was in this situation. He knew I was tired, in pain and depleted of patience. Why couldn't he work this out? With my head pounding and my emotional state shaky, I felt like God was against me, not for me. I felt like I was being tormented by him, not loved. As my walk continued, I voiced my disappointment with an honesty and audacity I don't normally attempt with God Almighty, but I didn't care. He had to hear me out.

My monologue covered the details from my decades of dealing with these blasted headaches, the hundreds of prayers I had spoken, the road construction he could have changed, and how he was failing me. How long did he expect my hope to last? How many prayers would be enough? How did he expect me to believe in him and his supposed love for me when he never offered any relief? Where was his compassion? He knew my situation and had the power to change it. "Come on already, BE GOD!" I cried.

Then I thought of the millions of people worse off than I—images of the starving, war-torn, homeless, the terminal patients who were undoubtedly crying out for help flashed in my mind. The high death rate and lack of miraculous healings scared me. If God doesn't save the starving children or the mother of four dying with cancer, why in the world would he help me with my headaches? The world situation didn't seem to reflect a loving God in charge. Shoot, maybe he wasn't.

I wiped my face with my bare arm and started kicking a stone in front of me. As my walk continued, I remembered a Bible story about Jesus healing a leper. The leper falls on his face in front of Jesus and says, "Lord, if you are willing, you can make me clean."[8] I pictured the leper lying on his face in front of Jesus, desperate for healing and was challenged by his humility and willingness to give God the option of healing him or not. I knew I wasn't at the point of giving God options. All I wanted was God to do what I wanted him to do! I wondered about the leper's faith. I wondered about mine.

The leper, physically suffering and socially isolated because of his disease, was allowing God to *choose* whether or not to heal him while fully believing he could if he wanted to. His faith is deep with reverence, trust, and submissiveness. I realized mine wasn't.

The story goes on to tell Jesus' response: "I am willing; be cleansed."[9] Of course God is willing. But then why doesn't he always answer the broken-hearted crying out for help and healing in the affirmative? The story offered no relief, and I kicked the stone in front of me down the street drain.

Broken as I was, I remembered the garbage men. As I walked, they kept passing me. I wondered if they were really picking up garbage or just driving by out of curiosity. There was nowhere to hide, so I looked straight ahead and kept crying as the heat rising up from the black asphalt road burned my face.

At mid-morning, this neighborhood was quiet, allowing me to hear my footsteps, the noise of all the moisture dripping out of my eyes and nose, and each rustle of the leaves on the side of the street. I heard someone opening their garage door and the crows cawing up above me. Then there were those dumb cicada bugs with their noisy, rhythmic, buzzing that made the moment feel especially desperate. Each time the garbage men drove by, I felt their eyes on me. I could only imagine what they were thinking, and, somewhere deep inside, it made me grin and turn back to find Mike and Grace.

When I returned, my husband was busily rearranging his work schedule and the kids so that I could make this later appointment. I recall just sitting there in our family's van, depleted of energy, understanding, and grace as Mike called colleagues, courtrooms, neighbors and judges to allow me this later time. It would've been easier for him if he just had to cancel some client appointments or miss time in the office, but he had a court appearance in the afternoon. Lawyers usually don't call judges and tell them they can't make it, but Mike did. I had definitely hit bottom and didn't know what else to do but sit there and let him do it.

As Mike rallied, Grace sat on my lap smothering me with kisses I didn't want. I couldn't return the emotion. I could barely wrap my arm around her. She kissed and hugged me over and over again, whispering "I love you" in my ear until her face was covered with my tears. She continued wet and undeterred while I just sat there letting her.

We then went to lunch. I was numb and unable to speak without crying. The food smelled delicious, but didn't rouse my appetite, and, although I noticed the concerned looks passing between the waitress, Grace, and my husband, I was unmoved. It had been a long road here with too many painful days. I think that morning was the first time I fully let myself acknowledge all that I dealt with year after year, and my body broke in grief over the whole thing.

There was no escaping the current nightmare in my head, and I wanted to scream at the heavens, "Where are you? Why won't you help me and stop this crazy head of mine from hurting? What kind of Savior are you anyway?"

I felt utterly helpless and abandoned by this God I loved most of my life. Mike recognized my fragile state and just hovered ready to help in any way. I'm not sure how I would have made it through that day without his physical presence. There are days when those around you need to drop everything just for you. I am glad he did.

As I have told this story to others, I have found myself discussing a particular Bible verse promising that God will not give us more than we can handle:

> No temptation has overtaken you that is not common to man. God is faithful, and he will not let you be tempted beyond your ability, but with the temptation he will also provide the way of escape, that you may be able to endure it.[10]

I suppose I never had that verse right. It doesn't read that God will spare us from anything we can't handle, but, rather, God will provide *a way of escape* so that we will be able to endure. Very different and much less appealing than my version.

I always felt safeguarded by that verse when I thought it meant that God would never give me more than I could handle. I believed I couldn't handle much trouble, so he wouldn't allow much trouble to enter my life. I knew my weakness and believed God wouldn't allow a tragedy to befall me, knowing full well I couldn't stand it. I didn't possess the faith of Job, the bravery of Joan of Arc, or the wit and wisdom of Benjamin Franklin. I am weak and always counted on that fact to protect me from great pain and calamity.

With this new understanding, fear rose in me—a fear that my troubles and pain would one day exceed the realm of headaches, migraines, and other sundry messes of life. I pushed the thoughts and fear away, unable to digest this new truth—the truth that anything bad can happen to any of us at any time. After a lifetime of believing that God protected me from devastation and horror, I realized his promise wasn't about sparing us; it was about providing a way to endure.

So, if the safeguard wasn't there, where was my escape? I suppose he was sitting across the table from me ordering the lunch special and a Coca-Cola. What would the day have looked like if I had driven myself to the appointment? Mike doesn't usually join me for headache appointments. This was the first and only time he came along. I can say it was one of a few days in my life where I could feel something inside me break. I think when you hold on to hope and endure something for a long time, there are days when you just let go and all you can do is grieve.

On my walk that morning, I cried out to God, asking him where he was in my pain. Not only did he feel far away, but he also didn't appear to want to help me. He could've made the morning work. A little tweak here and there with the morning preparations and the road construction problem, and we would have made it. Why did he allow it to happen? Why couldn't he soften the receptionist's heart?

But in my hour of crumbling, Mike had the get-away van along with Grace ready to whisk me out of that parking lot and off to Maureen's diner. It actually was enough to help me endure.

There were hours between lunch at Maureen's and my afternoon appointment. Mike paid our bill, and I couldn't help but notice again the sympathetic glances he and the waitress exchanged. I hoped he tipped her well. Mike carried Grace to the van and buckled her up. I climbed into the passenger's seat, shut the door, and stared out the window. Leaving the parking lot, my mind began to wander.

I remembered a phone call from the previous week with a friend of mine currently living a nightmare. She had three small, needy children, and her husband was a drug addict. She was raised by an alcoholic mother and made it her life's goal never to live with an addict again. She married her husband, who, at surface level, seemed to have all that she wanted and none of what she feared. After three children together, she came to find that her seemingly stable and successful man couldn't get through the day without drinking, and she wondered how she could possibly be in that situation. She believed in God and had prayed at every turn for guidance. What did she miss? How could her Savior not have saved her from this?

During our conversation, we wondered about that question. We looked back over the last few years and saw that God didn't save her from marrying a man with an addiction but seemed to be providing along the way to help her endure.

We remembered how her once addicted mother has been sober for years and is a source of love, support, and inspiration. Her father also adores her and they are both fantastic grandparents who love her three babies. We remembered how they once lived thousands of miles away but now lived nearby. Near enough to help her. As awful as her situation was, God seemed to be providing for her in the midst of her struggle.

Our remembering didn't seem to lift her spirits much. I hung up the phone, fully realizing my ability to see God's involvement and love in her life was because of my pain-free vantage point. I'm not the one living with three little ones, fearing what will walk through the door at the end of the day. I prayed that her troubles would resolve themselves quickly.

I have prayed the quick, poof-be-gone prayer one too many times to think that those situations, personalities, and consequences are likely to disappear into thin air. But I can't seem to give up on the idea that if I pray, God will make all the bad supernaturally disappear. I so desperately want the pain I pray for to end quickly whether it's mine or someone else's. I guessed her road might continue hard, long and winding, and, in the end, look nothing like I imagined or hoped. I trusted that whatever the ending was for her and her family, it would be *better* than my prayer requests—a deeper, wider resolution brought about over time.

Maybe I should pray differently—more for her along the road than for an instantaneous, miraculous solution.

Sometimes we are the cause of our own pain. It's easy to blame God for the pain in our lives even when we are the ones who made the bad choices along the way—whether consciously or naively—ignoring God's wisdom and even his commandments that were meant to spare us from so much misery. It sounds harsh, but it's true.

Other times, I've fallen victim to other people's choices. Their greed or selfishness affects our businesses, livelihoods, 401K's, and our children's futures. Many of us have grown up around alcoholics who have poisoned Christmas celebrations and turned many a night into tormenting worry as we wait for the inevitable to happen.

And sometimes pain is a result of an illness, disability, or accident. Events we never saw coming that change our lives in a moment. We are undeserving, unprepared, and devastated by the uncontrollable, unpredictable happenings of this world. Our lives change instantly, and, in shock, we stagger through days wondering when it will be over.

Or we choose a different response to the pain.

We exercise our free will and consciously choose not to be destroyed by it, even though it continually tempts and taunts us to surrender in defeat.

I have witnessed lives who have suffered more than I can or want to imagine and have watched them stumble without falling. Their fight and resolve fill me with hope and wonder. What do they know that I can't yet see or understand? How has God provided an escape for them? *They* are the ones who hold the key to pain and suffering. They are wounded but sustained; humbled but strong; sobered but still able to know joy. Amazing people I want to emulate.

Whatever the case may be, I realize none of us are immune or safeguarded from any of it. The promise seems to be that God can meet us *in the pain* and provide whatever we need to survive. We are not guaranteed safe passage to heaven's shores. Most likely, we will all arrive worn out, bloody from battle, tested, tried, and refined by the fires of life. There is no protection from pain, tragedy, death, and devastation. Perhaps the fact that we *can* arrive at heaven's shores should be our focus and, in the end, our ultimate escape. Maybe.

Our ride home was certainly quicker than our ride there. Mike found a faster detour around the road construction and soon we were pulling into our driveway. Grace was asleep and Mike carefully carried her to her bedroom while I crawled into my own bed. I had a couple of hours before I had to return to the doctor's office. Mike would be staying home with the kids for the rest of the day, having worked out his schedule, and when the new appointment time neared, I would head back by myself. I fell asleep.

Years ago, now, some friends of ours had the most unthinkable tragedy happen. They lost their eighteen-year-old son in a horrible car accident. I think of them and wonder how they are able to get out of bed, talk, go food shopping, breathe, and watch a day begin and end. My heart breaks and aches for them. How can this not be too much for a parent to bear? How can a mother say goodbye to her son? How can a dad lose his boy and survive? Why would God allow it?

A year later at a memorial weekend for their son, I watched them. They were broken but breathing. They were in grief, and yet I witnessed them enjoying good conversation and even a laugh with friends. Their other children were running and playing, and they were all lovingly surrounded by family.

I watched, wondering where they found the will to go on and the strength to get through the days. I know their journey has been more difficult than I can fathom and am sure there are many dark days behind and ahead of them. I sat near them in church, and I could hear them singing. Singing. As I strained to listen to their voices, I was confounded by their staying power and humbled in their presence. I listened in awe as their voices gently, weakly sang a song. There must be a God if they can whisper a song of hope after their son's death. There must be someone else holding them up and loving them—a power stronger than the pain.

Crushed, but not destroyed.

They weren't running from their pain or masking it with drugs and denial. They were living the pain and finding their way through their days with friends, family, and God. When I talked to the mom, I felt her open wound and listened intently as she spoke of her inconceivable loss with peace, hope, anger, bewilderment, sweetness, despair, frailty, and strength. It was all there wrapped up in one living, breathing mother who was still standing, still holding on. I could sense that there was something greater sustaining her as she walked through the "valley of the shadow of death."[11]

My situation doesn't compare. Why do I only have chronic head pain while someone else endures the loss of a child? Why do some of us live with plenty while others die of hunger? Why did some survive the accident while others perished? I have no clue. But in the tragedies, illnesses, accidents, and deaths I have seen evidence of more. More than our physical circumstances. More than our ability to survive. More power than the pain. More than we can see with our eyes and touch with our hands.

I woke up to Mike's face hovering above mine, whispering that it was time for me to leave. How was I going to drive back to the doctor's office by myself feeling so miserable? I sat on the edge of my bed, trying to gather strength and desire. Finally, with a little of both, I got my body out the door and back into the car. Mike stood at the front door, watching, and I could see his sympathy for me on his face. I put on my sunglasses, adjusted the rear-view mirror, and took a deep breath. Exhaling my millionth "God help me," I stepped on the gas pedal and drove away.

While driving, I recalled a verse that reads: "And we know that for those who love God all things work together for good, for those who are called according to his purpose."[12] But, when the pain persists and even grows it certainly doesn't seem like "all things worked together for good." It actually looks like all things worked together to create the worst-case scenario.

Perhaps I have never understood that reference either. Perhaps God's definition of good is different from mine. Perhaps he is willing to let anything happen to us because he knows there is not a place—no matter how dark or deep—he cannot come and keep us company, not a pit he won't sit in by our side, not a road he is not willing to walk with us. Maybe God wants us stripped and helpless, desperate, lying in a heap at his feet crying for deliverance, so he can truly deliver us—not in a physical sense, but something much greater. Lord, have mercy.

I put on my blinker and made the left onto the highway entrance. As I merged into the traffic and wove my van across three lanes and then back over two settling in behind a Porsche going eighty miles an hour, I realized I better calm down. I decreased my speed to sixty-five and continued the thought process.

What if we surrendered to God's ways? What if we didn't become embittered, but obedient and compliant? What if we didn't run from him in our despair, but fell into his arms, helpless and needing comfort? What if we didn't let our fear rule the day but, rather, trusted him in the darkness? What if we had no hope but him and stood face to face with God and just waited for him to do something with us, for us. Immovable until he moved us. What would he do? What would he say?

I remembered listening to Reverend Billy Graham speak on television at the National Cathedral in Washington D.C. on September 14, 2001, after the terrorists had attacked our nation. My community was reeling in grief as we were forced to digest the fact that some of our friends would never return home from work. The odor in our suburban air was a constant, awful reminder that New York was burning, and people were dead. With dread and a fearful spirit, I sat on the edge of the chair in our family room, staring at the television, ready to drink in a word of encouragement from a man I admired and trusted. He read the following from the book of Psalms:

> God is our refuge and strength, a very present help in
> trouble.
> Therefore we will not fear though the earth gives way,
> though the mountains be moved into the heart of the
> sea,

though its waters roar and foam, though the mountains
tremble at its swelling.
There is a river whose streams make glad the city of
God, the holy habitation of the Most High.
God is in the midst of her; she shall not be moved; God
will help her when morning dawns.
The nations rage, the kingdoms totter; he utters his
voice, the earth melts.
The LORD of hosts is with us; the God of Jacob is our
fortress…
"Be still, and know that I am God. I will be exalted
among the nations, I will be exalted in the earth!"
The LORD of hosts is with us; the God of Jacob is our
fortress.[13]

As Reverend Graham closed his Bible, I concluded that God seems to allow the horrible to happen. The only phrase in that passage that is repeated by the writer is "The Lord of hosts is with us." Usually, when there is a repeat in literature, it means it's important. So, I dwelled on the fact that though God allows "the mountains to slip into the heart of the sea," he promises to be with us in our trouble and not leave us alone to fend for ourselves.

I pulled into the doctor's parking lot for the second time that day, thinking that somehow his presence has got to be enough to sustain me. I supposed the hard part was figuring out how to know and experience "God with us" to the extent that it actually helps.

To get to that point in the hardest trials or most painful of circumstances seems impossible. How do you keep company and embrace a God that allowed the horrible to happen? How do you love the Lord of hosts when every day you pray for relief from your pain, and it is not granted? If we could quickly exhale in surrender and inhale his presence how would our situation change? I can hear Billy Graham's voice reading, "Be still, and know that I am God…" Perhaps that's the key.

Opening the door to the waiting room, I was stunned by the crowd. I suppose canceling my morning appointment didn't help their overbooked schedule much. Stepping over children playing on the floor, I checked in without making eye contact with the receptionist and found a seat in the only available chair.

I released an unusually heavy sigh and thought of Job from the Old Testament. His life tells a story of incomprehensible suffering and faith. In this historical passage, Satan thinks that God's faithful servant Job is "a blameless and upright man, who fears God and turns away from evil"[14] only because God has put a hedge of protection around him and blessed him with great wealth. But God, sure of Job's faith in him, allows Satan to test Job in any way as long as he doesn't kill him. At this allowance, Satan departs from the presence of the Lord and begins his assault.

During the first day, Job loses his livestock, servants, seven sons, and three daughters. When the surviving servants delivered the bad news, Job "arose and tore his robe and shaved his head and fell on the ground and worshiped."[15] Worshiped? Are you kidding me?

> And he said, "Naked I came from my mother's womb, and naked shall I return. The Lord gave, and the Lord has taken away; blessed be the name of the Lord."[16]

Blessed be the name of the Lord? What kind of man after losing everything can say that? What does it say about him and his faith? What does it say about the God he serves? It is recorded that through all of his ordeal, "Job did not sin or charge God with wrong."[17] Astounding.

Remembering Job's story, I am struck by the fact that Job accepted God in all his holiness and sovereignty. He lived in complete submission to God's will. No questions asked. The Lord gives. The Lord takes away. Blessed be the name of the Lord.

Toward the end of the book, Job becomes more discouraged as his friends offer rebuke rather than comfort as Satan's assault continues. Ultimately, the Lord speaks out against Job's shameful friends. Job and his friends listen as the voice of the Lord bellows from a whirlwind crying,

> Who is this that darkens counsel by words without
> knowledge?
> Dress for action like a man;
> I will question you, and you make it known to me.
>
> Where were you when I laid the foundation of the
> earth?
> Tell me, if you have understanding.
> Who determined its measurements—surely you know?
> Or who stretched the line upon it?
> On what were its bases sunk,
> or who laid its cornerstone,
> when the morning stars sang together,
> and all the sons of God shouted for joy?[18]

I don't know about you, but I quiver at those words thundering from the mouth of God. I am humbled as I recall my numerous responses to pain or calamity that were filled with blame and bitterness as I questioned God Almighty. The Lord's might and power shut me right up and I realize it would serve me well to be still and know that He is God[19] more often than I do.

Ruminating on the death of my friend's son, 9/11, and the life of Job, I am reminded again of why I don't like to mention my migraines. But these headaches are the pain I know. I am grateful they are not more than they are while also burdened by their impact. My pain is what I have been given to deal with. I don't know why I wasn't given more, and I don't know why I wasn't given less. But I can say my headaches have served as my introduction to the pain that brews, boils, and languishes all over this world. They've opened my eyes and broken my heart, enabling me to catch a glimpse and begin to empathize with those suffering less along with those burdened with so much more. Without them, I couldn't relate on any level to the hurting world around me. I believe my headaches give me awareness and understanding—allowing me to care more than I would and love better than I could without them. So, that's a plus.

While waiting, I eavesdropped and learned that some of the patients traveled from out of state each month to see this particular doctor. Couldn't imagine waiting in this room once a month. Couldn't imagine driving in from out of state. "He must be good," I thought, trying to regain my hope and equilibrium. I occasionally glared at the receptionist (who was still smiling) and had bad thoughts. It took every ounce of self-control not to tap on her glass window and give her an earful.

My left shoulder was up against the gentleman seated next to me. He didn't seem bothered by the mass of people keeping us company or the wait, nor was he engrossed in a book or looking to strike up conversation (thank goodness). His calm demeanor sat in contrast to my agitated state as I flipped through magazines, keeping tabs on the cold-hearted receptionist. As minutes turned to hours, his steadiness rubbed off on me, and I eventually relaxed into a state of calm resignation. Under better circumstances I may have tried to start a conversation with the man, but I didn't, and I was thankful he didn't either.

Two and a half hours later, they called my name. Bitter, I peeled myself out of my seat and walked toward the receptionist waiting at the door. I made no eye contact and trudged down the hallway like a beaten prisoner. I entered the doctor's office and slumped down in the chair waiting for me across from his desk. At first sight, he must've thought I was in definite need of a doctor. My makeup was long cried off, and my face was blotchy. The bags under my eyes from the migraine were dark, and all my hair was greased back in a tight knot because I couldn't deal with it. I was miserable and exhausted. I stared at my lap and sat there, trying not to move my pounding head—waiting for his questions to begin.

He was obviously having a busy afternoon. He shuffled through his pile of papers looking for my information. I could sense him trying to shift gears from whatever his last appointment filled his mind with and refocus on the new one in front of him. He gave a stab at conversation, but my monosyllabic responses led to dead ends. Although he was trying to give me his all, I decided that no doctor should be as busy as he was. What human being can think straight after hours and hours of back-to-back appointments? He began his basic questioning about my health history, and I gave him the abridged version. Once he had completed my questionnaire, he started his testing using a special machine developed and widely used in Europe.

This time I was allowed to stay fully clothed and there were no needles in sight. My fingers were hooked up to a wire coming from a machine that would read my "levels" as I held glass vials of different substances in my hand. I held bottle after bottle of various foods, elements, vitamins, etc. Anything you could possibly be allergic to. I would hear the machine beep frantically for some vials and fall silent on others. The doctor took notes as we proceeded. It was a fascinating process and took my mind off my misery for a while.

Through electromagnetic energy, he said he could detect body weaknesses, allergies, and malfunctions. We could be here all day, I thought. I wondered if he'd pick up this morning's malfunction and start apologizing to me with regard to his unaccommodating receptionist. Not surprisingly, he finished with a long list of things that were wrong with my body, all of which he said we could address and fix.

At this point, I didn't buy that line anymore.

"We'll see," I told him. At the end of the session, he asked me how I heard of him. I told him a friend of mine knew numerous people at his church who were his patients and happy with the results. He nodded and then asked a question as he looked over my paperwork.

"Did you see the man sitting next to you in the waiting room?"

What kind of question is that? Of course I saw the man sitting next to me in the waiting room. For Pete's sake, we'd been sitting there for over two hours. I'm not blind and he certainly wasn't invisible. I kept my thoughts to myself, realizing I was still hostile and simply replied, "Yes, of course."

Then he said, "That was Jesus."

Oh, great. I've waited forever to see this doctor only to find out he's a total wacko. Letting out an awkward laugh, I looked for the exit door.

"He actually played the *role* of Jesus in the recent Easter play at your friend's church," he said.

Why would I care that the guy sitting next to me was in a church play as Jesus? It's not like it was a Broadway show or something worth mentioning. And when did the doctor peer into his crowded waiting room and take note of who was sitting next to whom? Did he have a peep hole in his office wall? Was I part of some "Candid Camera" television experiment? I mulled over my thoughts as he proceeded to give the nurse a list of things I would need to start the healing process. More supplements and diet restrictions. We shook hands, and I headed home.

That night after a hot shower, I curled up on our bed and ran through the day's events with Mike, thanking him for getting me through it.

"Do you think I'm absolutely nuts?" I asked.

"No, I think you're at the end of your rope, and I'm surprised it's taken you this long to get there. I feel terrible for you." He looked more wounded than I.

I talked about my morning thoughts about God and how I wondered where he was in this pain of mine. Mike didn't have an answer either. I told him each detail regarding my appointment from the two hour wait to the strange, electromagnetic machine, to the harried doctor, awful receptionist, and my complex, problematic body.

Then I mentioned the doctor's comment about Jesus sitting next to me in the waiting room and how I started to think the guy was some sort of nut job.

And it dawned on me.

In my exhaustion at the end of a horrible day, I got it, and if I hadn't spent half the day in tears, I think I would've started crying again.

Was it a coincidence that a man who played the role of Jesus was sitting next to me in the waiting room that day? Was it a coincidence that the doctor noticed him sitting next to me so that he could ask me about him? Was it a coincidence that my friends attended "Jesus'" church so that the doctor could even make that statement? Was it a coincidence that I was asking the question "Where are you, God?" throughout that long day? Some would say it was. Some days I would say it was.

But on this day, God couldn't have communicated his presence in a better, clearer way. "Jesus" was sitting right next to me in that awful waiting room for 2 ½ hours. God's answer to my question was clear: "I am always right next to you." That sentence along with my memory of "Jesus" that afternoon sitting shoulder to shoulder with me calming me down with his quietness pierced my heart. For reasons beyond my comprehension, God was choosing to sit next to me in my pain rather than deliver me from it. The pain suddenly seemed more bearable, if not altogether worthwhile.

The promise of God's presence was just that, a promise. I wondered how I could experience his presence in my pain to the degree where it would help me endure. For now, the adage "misery loves company" hung like a banner over my head, and I was grateful for his.

My season with this doctor was intense. It required discipline and deprivation that made my life difficult. Each visit pinpointed a particular substance in my diet that I was allergic to, and the following weeks required me to abstain from it, take the appropriate supplements, and return to his office and test to see if my body, as the doctor put it, cleared it. (Why these allergies didn't show up at the allergist's office eluded me.)

My desperation for relief made me do the work required and I was an outstanding patient…again. Each visit would clear me of the particular allergy, and we would move on to the next one. It was daunting to see the list of things that were having an adverse effect on my body. I am, in general, a healthy person who eats pretty well and exercises most of the time. It was hard to believe that my body was such a mess.

I thought of the many folks who live on fast food, don't exercise, and nary set foot in the fresh produce section of the supermarket and wondered why they weren't all plagued with headaches. The doctor tried to comfort me by saying everyone's system reacts differently to its environment and mine was very sensitive. No kidding.

At the end of six months, we made it through our list, and my body was supposedly allergy free. I drove to my last appointment with a searing headache. My faith in the process was shaky because my pain had persisted throughout, but I couldn't give up until it was finished. Perhaps it would be that last allergy that was causing all the trouble. So, I hung in there until my list was completed.

Once the last allergy cleared, I sat with my migraine thundering against my eyes, staring at the doctor across his cluttered desk, wondering what his next step would be. He concluded that I had a virus in my body that was not allowing the headaches to clear and we would have to spend the next few months trying to get rid of it.

I laid my head down on his desk to collect my thoughts. Instead of feeling my energy surge for our next attempt, I felt my hope slip. A proverb came to mind: "Hope deferred makes the heart sick."[20] I wanted to partner with the doctor and try his next attempt to solve my head pain, but my usual hope wasn't there. I realized my faith in him and his unique approach was gone, and I didn't believe him enough to continue. Slowly lifting my head up, I told him I couldn't do it.

So I left with my sick head and heart, bid good riddance to the receptionist, and departed from that particular waiting room, trusting Jesus would follow me out the door.

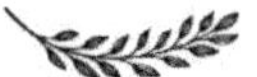

And behold, I am with you always, to the end of the age.

Matthew 28:20b, ESV

6

Is Anybody Listening?

Most days I come away with unfulfilled longings, unrequited initiatives, unanswered prayers, unrealized aspirations, deferred hopes and incomplete understandings. But then along comes one of those days ... when heaven leans over and God speaks a word directly to the heart.

—Bob Sorge[21]

DECIDING TO LET UP ON DOCTOR APPOINTMENTS for a while, I gladly entered into my routines without distraction. One of my better weekly commitments was a small study group that started meeting at my house years earlier to study the Bible and learn more about God. The group evolved into a community of friends over time, and I loved learning, growing, and praying alongside each one of them. We were always able to maintain a certain authenticity, and it became a comfortable place to share thoughts, questions, study, pray, and, out of sheer need or desire, laugh or cry.

Each of us represented a different perspective. We saw from a variety of vantage points, had unique educational and professional backgrounds, along with personalities that ran the gamut. But when Terry opened a meeting with her humble voice and reverent tone praying, "Our most gracious heavenly Father, Ruler of all things, and Lover of our souls, we adore you...", a hush covered the room and, despite our differences and the noise of the day, we were called to attention and keenly aware of what we were trying to do and who we were addressing.

After I made my decision to share my headache problem with others, this group of women was a natural place for me to start. During our meetings, we often prayed for each other, and they often prayed for me and my aching head. At one particular meeting, Jackie wanted to follow up on a few of our requests to see what God was doing. She wanted a report, wanted to know what she could check off her list as accomplished and done.

So, we went around the room and each person reported their rather dismal news. The broken relationship we had been praying for was more broken; the cancerous friend had died; the sick were still sick; and my head was still pounding. The room was silent after the inventory had been taken, and I didn't quite know what to say. "Well, ladies, keep up the good work! Anything else you would like us to pray for?" What do you do with all that bad news?

In desperation, someone asked about my lost red wallet that we had prayed about a couple of weeks ago, hoping for a *little* good news. I slowly replied that the red wallet was still lost; I had looked everywhere, and I was still delinquent (or lazy) enough to have not yet canceled my credit cards or secured a new driver's license. With that, we closed the meeting.

As I waved and watched their cars pull out of my driveway, I grew despondent over our praying track record. I felt badly for my friends who wanted positive answers to their serious requests. I thought of the friend who had died and the couple filing for divorce and was sad for them and their loved ones who had been praying for a better outcome. It was discouraging, and I couldn't help but wonder again if God was listening, and if so, why wasn't he healing the sick and restoring the broken?

I closed the front door and began the business of the day—which always seems to involve laundry. I thought I would chase away the bad feelings and disappointment through activity. Emptying all the laundry baskets, including the big one in the linen closet, I began the long process of cleaning my family's clothes.

As I bent over the tall basket, I chucked clothes up and out over my shoulders until it was emptied. My mind raced with the unanswered prayers, sad faces, and God's apparent indifference. Then as I hauled the last pair of dirty socks out of the bottom of the basket, there it was. I straightened up without taking my eyes off it—half thinking it might disappear again. I was frozen in place as my wallet and I just stared at each other. After weeks of hunting for it, having done plenty of laundry, how could it be at the bottom of this basket? Who could ignore the timing? It felt like God was trying to tell me something—perhaps that he *was* listening to our prayers. The moment was humbling. Even though I was tempted to continue the conversation and press him further as to why he wasn't answering our prayer requests according to our wishes, all of a sudden, I didn't feel the need. So I just stood there, staring at the red wallet in my hand, took a deep breath, and exhaled. I bowed my head in surrender—relinquishing my arguments and disappointments. And then relief and peace settled into my bones.

What will it take for me to respond to disappointment with trust, not doubt; acceptance and curiosity about what God is up to, instead of annoyance that he's not granting my prayer wishes? What will it take for me to remember that God is good even when I am surrounded by bad?

I think remembering is key. When I remember in my present pain, disappointment, confusion, or difficulty what God has done for me in the past, it bolsters my resolve to keep the faith and trust him despite my inability to see any reason, relief, sense, or explanation for the pain or bad circumstances. But it's hard to remember the past and our need to "keep the faith" *while* suffering. The suffering and pain overwhelm us like an ocean wave, and everything seems to get stripped away in the undertow …except what hurts. Although it would be helpful and possibly life-changing to live in a state of sustained remembrance, it's near impossible. But not completely.

So, I try to remember.

To remember other people's stories. To remember God knows what he is doing. To remember God is love. God is good. To remember he is with us. To remember this world is filled with trouble. To remember the lessons learned from the heartache. To remember we made it through nonetheless, because of grace and mercy and those we met along the way. To remember what you said you would never forget.

Easier said than done. We want to remember, but we simply forget.

I was finally done sorting out the laundry into various piles of whites, darks, and brights and stuck my red wallet in the back pocket of my jeans. Gathering an armload of darks, I made my way to the downstairs laundry room and swore I would remember this moment.

I then thought of the many references and techniques regarding "remembering" from the Bible—how to do it and why it's important. For instance, there's the story of how God gave Moses and the sons of Israel a song with lyrics describing every detail of the crossing of the Red Sea to help them remember what he did and how he saved them out of Egypt.[22] He didn't just want *them* to remember but their children and grandchildren too. The memories would fade; eyewitnesses would eventually die, but a song could be passed along forever.

It amazes me how I can still recite the lyrics to old 70's songs I listened to on my FM radio during my junior high school years. Is there really any advantage to knowing every last word to "Muskrat Love?" I hated that song, and I still know the words. And when I am in a hymn-singing crowd, I can go at least three verses deep into an old church hymn that I heard year after year sitting in a pew with my parents. Songs are good tools for remembering.

As the Israelites wandered their way through the desert on their way to the promised land, they must have sung songs of remembrance over and over again. The Song of Moses. When the sand got hot, the company tiresome, the manna monotonous, and the walking arduous, I can imagine them lifting up the Song of Moses again and again, helping them remember all God had done for them and, in so doing, regaining their hope and resolve to keep going.

Then there was Joshua's pile of stones that he stacked up after the Israelites had miraculously crossed over the Jordan River.[23] What a great way to memorialize the event and help them remember what God had done. And they *would* remember every time they saw the sacred pile of rocks. Every time a child pointed at it and asked what it was for, they would remember again.

I crammed the washer full of clothes, hoping I wasn't rendering the machine ineffective. My mind wandered to my last encounter with stone monuments while on a family trip to Gettysburg, Pennsylvania. Mike, the kids, and I were on our way to a lacrosse tournament for our oldest son, Matt, and figured a little history along the way wouldn't be the worst idea. I had never gone as a kid and had no idea what to expect. As we crested the hill and the Civil War battlefield spread out on either side of our truck, I was shocked. I had no idea they preserved the entire battlefield. It was acres and acres of beautiful farmland littered with majestic marble statues and monuments memorializing all who had died in these fields. The contrast of the monuments nestled in the natural landscape was vivid. Not a soul on earth could possibly drive down this country road without pulling over to ask, "What happened here?" Memorials are effective tools for remembering, and my family learned more in a day than we had in a long while. It was good to remember. And the next time I heard the national anthem, I choked up with emotion. Remembering is powerful stuff.

Pouring the detergent, I trusted the washer to do its work and went to the kitchen to make a cup of tea. I waited for the water to boil and then allowed the tea bag to steep for the required three minutes. Grabbing a seat in the kitchen I continued with my thoughts. Why in the Old Testament did God command his people to diligently teach his commandments to their sons, to talk of them when they were in their houses, out walking, when they were lying down and getting up? I recalled the passage where the Israelites were instructed to bind God's commandments as a sign on their hands and put bands on their foreheads. They were to write them on the doorposts of their houses and on their gates.[24] It seems to me that God was definitely concerned with their ability to remember his teachings.

Sometimes I think it would do me well to write God's instructions on my body and paint them on my doorposts. Perhaps we could put the current tattooing craze to better use? Taking a long sip of my tea, I stared out the window to my front porch, wondering what the doors and posts would look like painted with God's commandments. Interesting idea.

And then there's the Holy Spirit. In the book of John, it says, "But the Helper, the Holy Spirit, whom the Father will send in my name, he will teach you all things and bring to your remembrance all that I have said to you."[25] Thank goodness. Sometimes I can't remember what I did yesterday. I finished my tea grateful that God gave us his Spirit to help remind us of everything. Such a great idea.

I need all kinds of reminders of how God has worked in my past to get me through the present as I try to live by faith and believe that God will somehow deliver me. I believe that God calls us to "remember" over and over again in the Scriptures because he knows we are forgetful. Can you imagine the Israelites, after being delivered from slavery in Egypt with great drama and mighty acts of God, after crossing the Red Sea on a dry seabed with a wall of water roaring on either side of them, after they sang songs of praise and danced about with joy at how God had miraculously saved them, started grumbling because they were thirsty and hungry? Just days after God's miraculous parting of the Red Sea, they were filled with despair and hopelessness, not believing that the God who saved them from the Egyptians could also satisfy their hunger and thirst. They groaned, "Oh, if we could only go back to Egypt where there is food and water" and "Oh, I can't believe we've been brought out to this wilderness to die" and "Oh, if we could only go back to slavery and sit by our pots of meat and eat bread to the full."[26]

When reading about the Israelites, it's clear how alike we are. Without remembering my past and what God has done, I forget that he has proven himself faithful, and I fall into the same trap of grumbling and unbelief. But when I think back and remember an unexpected friend showing up just in time, a word of encouragement spoken exactly when needed, grace bestowed, protection unseen, and needs met—over and over again, I am reminded of God's faithfulness. Reflecting on the specifics of my life—who showed up when and what carried me through—I am humbled and overwhelmed by God's subtle and sometimes not so subtle provision. Taking inventory of my life leads me back to God. I should do it more often. I loaded my teacup along with the rest of the dirty dishes into the dishwasher and headed back to the laundry room to check the progress.

The darks went into the dryer, and I loaded the whites, adding a shot of bleach to the detergent. It is so satisfying having machines do your dirty work. I closed the laundry room door and headed back to the kitchen to prep food for dinner. Deciding to take my own advice and do some remembering, I thought back to the day I was baptized.

I remember it well. I was up at a camp in New Hampshire where I spent my summers as a kid. Second to my childhood church, summers at this Christian camp most deeply impacted my belief in God—whether it was the Bible stories, campfire songs, the camp counselors who prayed with me, or just the beautiful surroundings that naturally grabbed my attention making me wonder about a Creator. It was a strong influence. Getting baptized in that lake just seemed right to me, and so, after a summer working as a camp counselor, I thought it was time. I was twenty-one years old, full of faith, wanting to publicly testify that I belonged to Jesus.

After chapel on an August Sunday morning, I went down to the beach with the congregation. Two of my good friends were also being baptized, and we made our way to the shoreline while everyone else stood looking on. When it came my turn, I requested the hymn "Great Is Thy Faithfulness" to be sung before my body got dunked in the name of the Father, Son, and Holy Ghost. I loved the lyrics and knew even then they were true. Everyone on the beach sang it for me while I waited waist deep in water soaking in every word. As my voice joined with theirs, I thought of the many times I sang that song while driving with my father on road trips, how the words had been written on my heart, and how I knew they would hold true 'til the day I died. There are moments in life when you just know. The day I got baptized I knew how great God's faithfulness was and is and always will be. I can still hear those voices rising from the beach singing:

> Great is Thy faithfulness, O God, My Father.
> There is no shadow of turning with Thee.
> Thou changest not, Thy compassions they fail not.
> As Thou hast been, Thou forever will be.
>
> Great is Thy faithfulness.
> Great is Thy Faithfulness.
> Morning by morning new mercies I see.
> All I have needed, Thy hand hath provided.
> Great is Thy faithfulness, Lord unto me.[27]

I started humming the song as I smashed the ground meats together and added the breadcrumbs and seasonings. We were having meatballs for dinner. I felt invigorated as I rolled the meat into balls now singing "Great Is Thy Faithfulness" in full voice. Remembering is good.

I resolved yet again to try and remember my past and be patient when I offer prayers to God and hear nothing or, worse yet, hear "no." Maybe God's answer is in the waiting. Maybe when he doesn't respond to my prayers to heal my aching head, it's because he wants me to know there's more to this spiritual life than getting my pain relieved. Maybe there are benefits that can only be found in suffering, treasures buried in the pain that he wants me to find—kind of like my wallet under all that laundry.

One of my favorite things to do as a child was listen to stories my dad would tell about his father. Knowing faithful people and hearing stories of their faith-filled lives helps build, well, faith—at least for me. My grandfather was one of those people whose faith strengthened mine.

My grandfather died when he was ninety-two, but I remember his knowing eyes and soft smile. His usual expression of deep contentment both put me at ease and made me curious as a kid. I can still picture his nodding head, closed eyes, and how he would punctuate your words with "yeses" as he listened intently during conversations—making you say more than you planned. I don't think I have ever met anyone more faithful and humble than he.

He usually dressed in neat trousers, a sport coat or cardigan sweater, tie, and oftentimes, a hat. His manner was meek and thoughtful; sure, but unimposing; serious, but not stern; morally grounded, but never judgmental. He was easy with the young and the old, the down and out or society folk, believers and atheists. He never drew attention to himself and lived his life out in the background, not center stage—unless, of course, he was preaching.

In his early twenties, he lived far from his home in Norway, working as a mason in Chicago, trying to make money that couldn't be made at home. While in Chicago, he was "saved" (as he put it) at an evangelistic meeting. Having heard and believed in this "gospel of grace, forgiveness, and salvation," he swore he would never be the same. He returned to Norway when he had enough savings to get married and start a family, promising himself to tell anyone willing to listen about Jesus.

His experience in America drew him to the local church in Norway where he became an elder and attended with my grandmother and their four children—their only son, my father. My dad remembers that no matter how busy life on the farm was, his father never started the day without prayer. Never. He also never missed a chance to talk to someone about their faith or, if asked, preach on Sunday mornings. During World War II, their church opened its doors six nights a week in response to the community's desire for more. Needless to say, my grandfather had many opportunities to share the good news of God's forgiveness and salvation.

I've listened to stories involving my grandfather's faith, and they give me hope and stir up my own. I remember one that took place on a Sunday. My father was around ten years old and recalled how his dad was preaching that morning at church while also planning to baptize fifteen people. It was a big day for their small, country congregation. My grandmother was setting the breakfast table that Sunday morning as the rain poured down.

My grandfather came into the kitchen after finishing his morning chores and told my grandmother, their three daughters, and my dad to eat breakfast without him. He was concerned about the weather, and they all knew he was going back to his bedroom to pray. He asked them to pray too. Sundays were always filled with prayer at their house, but this day my grandfather had a specific petition.

The Sunday service was planned for one o'clock and was going to take place outside the church building by the river for the baptisms. My grandfather knew if the rain didn't stop, the outdoor service would have to be canceled along with the baptisms. Even though it seemed like you could always reschedule, my grandfather seemed set on the day. He had an urgency about him when it came to spiritual things. He went to his bedroom to ask God to simply stop the rain. That was around 8:30 in the morning.

Right before the noon hour, my grandfather emerged brimming with a quiet confidence and told the family to grab the umbrellas for the long walk to church. My father couldn't believe they were going to walk the miles to church in the pouring rain for a service that would most likely need to be canceled. Regardless, they all made their way through the mud and weather.

A worried church elder caught sight of my dad's family coming down the road and ran out to greet my grandfather, explaining that there was no end in sight for the storm, and it didn't look like things were going to work out for the day. Once they all got inside the church, the frantic elder suggested that they pray. It was 12:45 p.m.

My grandfather kindly replied that he already prayed, and God said it was going to be okay. Just like that. Plain and simple.

My grandfather then led the crowd out of the church into the rain. My father thought he was crazy, but by the time they reached the river's edge, the rain had stopped, and before the first person was baptized, the sun was actually shining.

The congregation watched everyone get baptized, heard their testimonies of faith, listened to my grandfather preach, and then sang songs in the sunshine. My father told me that the long walk home was a joyful one. He remembered grabbing his father's hand in excitement over what had just happened, and my grandfather turned winking at him without a word as they sloshed their way back home, unable to stop smiling.

Once back inside their house, the rain started again. My father remembered being disappointed and turning to his dad to complain about how the rain had started again, to which my grandfather replied, "God only promised good weather for the service."

Things like this happened all the time with my grandfather. My dad said living with him made it easy to believe in God. My father recounted how the next day the village newspaper reported the terrible weather that had covered the region that day. It was also reported that my dad's small town had strangely experienced an afternoon of sun despite the deluge all around it. I believe my grandfather saved that article for years.

Listening to stories like that strengthen my belief that God still answers prayer and intervenes in our lives. My grandfather reminds me to pray boldly, believe without ceasing, and to trust God no matter what is happening around you. Even if it's pouring outside and God promised sunshine, believe. Believing in things unseen is a challenge, at least for me. How can we be certain of something we cannot see? How can we be sure of what we hope for? For me, the stories help.

I don't know why God engages with us in our circumstances or why he wants us to ask for things he already knows we need. Perhaps it's how God teaches. Maybe it's how he brings us into relationship with him. Actually, I'm pretty sure that's it.

So, why does God seem silent sometimes? Why does he answer negatively to a desperate request? When I think back over my life and prayers through the years, there are many prayers I am grateful he did not answer according to my desire. I realize God actually knows better than I do. He has higher thoughts and different ways of accomplishing what he wants to accomplish. The longer I live, the more I see this truth.

There are also requests that he has granted me, but not in my timing. With the gift of perspective, his timing has always proven better.

Then there are those pleas and requests that have gone unanswered much to my surprise and disappointment. I am forced to surrender to God in his sovereignty and sit with my loss—holding tight to this blind faith. My grip gets sore in the process, and when I can barely hold on, along comes a good story, a faith filled memory, an answered prayer, comfort, a companion for the road, or a supernatural moment that sweeps over me and the believing becomes easier again.

We are called to faith whether we understand what is happening or not. It is believing in things you cannot see or comprehend, a trust that transcends our circumstances. I always wonder if my faith in God will survive a season of great calamity and grief. Is my believing in these things I cannot see strong enough? Enduring chronic pain the size of a migraine is one thing, receiving a devastating diagnosis is a whole other level of suffering. Would I continue to believe God when I am faced with my worst nightmare?

Recently, my family attended two funerals. They were both men in their early fifties who attended our church, living lives sold out to the cause of Christ. One gentleman (in every sense of that word) was a successful businessman leading a life worthy of emulation—a good steward, a servant's heart, and true worshiper of God.

On any given Sunday, his able fingers moved around his guitar while his calm voice and gentle spirit invited us to look upward and worship. I watched in dismay as his beautiful wife and four children greeted each mourner with grace and dignity.

Then there was Jack. He attended our church too, and although I didn't know him, I felt compelled to attend the service just to let his grieving wife know that people care, even strangers. I sat through his service listening to his college buddy and friend of thirty years describe Jack's adventurous life and joy in living. He was a bike rider, snowboarder, hiker, pilot, wakeboarder, family guy, and financier whose latest venture and life goal was to stop world hunger. His business partner from London eloquently described Jack's imagination, intelligence, and drive that made his latest desire completely viable.

But despite the prayers following his motorcycle wreck, Jack's head-injured body never came out of the coma, and God took him home. Who can make sense of it? Why wouldn't God allow two fathers with years ahead of them, filled with great desire to do God's will on earth, to survive the illness and accident?

Not long ago I attended a women's conference on faith and listened to a mother tell how her nine-year-old son was killed by a car while riding his bike to deliver something to his sister at a friend's house. I physically covered my ears at points as she spoke because I found it unbearable. But, there she was explaining her pain and grief with tears falling down her face while simultaneously talking of God's peace and faithfulness. Astounding. She was living my worst nightmare and she still loved Jesus. Somehow in her grief she felt God's presence, and it was sustaining her.

As I listened, I was encouraged by God's obvious presence in her life as she told her story, but I also grieved that I have a God who allows his children to suffer so. As my history with God builds and I listen to the many stories of faith while living my own, I am learning—slowly learning—that just because God allows suffering, it doesn't mean he's the author of it. It doesn't mean his heart isn't broken alongside ours. And it certainly doesn't mean that he is going to allow us to suffer alone. He seems to show up in story after story keeping company with the brokenhearted, comforting those in grief, and somehow, in time, causing some sort of beauty to rise from the ashes. It's a miracle.

Knowing God listens to our prayers is somewhat encouraging, but if he doesn't answer our cries for healing, why bother? How do we pray? Why pray at all when God's gonna do what God's gonna do? Why keep asking for relief when his answer appears to be "no?"

I remember sitting in a hospital room praying like I never prayed before for a 12-year-old boy who was in a serious accident at our church's youth retreat. For whatever reason, I was alone with him for a long time and pleaded with God for his life, fully believing God could heal him. There were hundreds, if not thousands of people praying for Zach as I did. But, he died.

A few months later, a teenage girl from our church ran her car into a telephone pole. Her internal damage was extensive, and she was in intensive care for weeks with people again praying around the clock. Numerous times she slipped away, and her heart stopped beating. And just when all hope was lost, she improved. On her way home from the hospital, her car passed the church. Friends and family gathered in the church parking lot and waited for her car to arrive. There were hundreds of people who loved Sequoyah, who had prayed for her and were now overjoyed to welcome her home and celebrate her miraculous recovery. With balloons in hand, everyone went wild as her car pulled into the lot and she stepped out to greet everyone.

"The Lord gives, and the Lord takes away,"[28] my grandfather would have said.

I think I need to modify my approach to prayer a bit. I will continue to pray and ask God for anything and everything because the Bible tells us that we should, but once I am done with my petition, I want God to respond with his answer. I really have to stop telling God what to do, stop being so demanding and specific. I need to give God room to act and move in anyway he wants, trusting he is good and, well, smarter than me. In the end, we have to let God be God whether the outcomes to our prayers make sense or not. I'm guessing in time they will.

I remember how Jesus taught his disciples to pray: "Our Father in heaven, hallowed be Your name. Your kingdom come. Your will be done on earth as it is in heaven…"[29] A far more difficult prayer to say and mean than I realized.

I know God invites us to voice our needs and present our requests before him, but I also believe he wants us to keep praying even when the healing doesn't come—as hard as that is. And when I push through the disappointment of "unanswered prayers," stay on my knees, and keep talking to him, I see there's more to talk about—more to know than just freedom from pain, discomfort, and suffering. Much more.

When life is calm and disaster free, the good season lulls me into thinking that I can handle life quite well on my own. I get a couple of weeks without a headache, and my desperate body gets off its knees and starts to believe that I am alright without him. Really. I could go for a month with a headache, begging for mercy and relief through the days, but when relief appears, within a couple of days, I dump him. I don't do it consciously, but I drift away. There are words from an old church hymn that come to mind:

> Prone to wander, Lord, I feel it.
> Prone to leave the God I love…[30]

That would be me. My gratefulness turns to forgetfulness, and I am back to living my life without The One who created me. Although I might be pain free, it's never better and always lacking.

My painful days are spent by his side in constant conversation. When you spend that much time with God, you get to know him. Your spirit is in touch with his. You listen for him and he speaks. You see more than the physical world around you and become sensitive to the spiritual world—God's quiet whisper, how he reveals himself in nature, through people, the Bible, and circumstances. When I am forced to slow down because of my pain and grab hold of Him in my desperation, he is there. Without the pain, I seem to run around like a joyful lunatic only able to squeeze in a brief mealtime prayer and one more at bedtime. However, when I am confronted with grief, disaster, or pain, I fall back on my knees. In pain, I do not know what else to do or who else to turn to but God. In pain, I live each day with Jesus. Without the pain, I forget. Maybe that's the purpose of *my* pain—to bring and keep me by his side. If only I could learn to stay there without it. Maybe one day I will, and these headaches will finally stop.

Joni Eareckson Tada, who became a quadriplegic as a young girl after a devastating diving accident, states, "God always seems bigger to those who need Him most. And to be intimate with the Savior is to wake up in the morning needing Him desperately."[31] I suppose God is more desperate for us to know him well than for us to be pain free. Why would we turn to God if we didn't feel we needed a god? Without some sort of pain, it is hard to recognize our need, our need for someone to save us.

As God brings each one of us to that point of recognition in a million different ways, we have an opportunity to hold out our helpless hands and tired hearts and say "yes" to the One who longs to be a part of our lives. And although he may not heal us or deliver us from our pain and trouble, he promises to listen, to love, and be near. He promises to save us—not from our present pain, but from eternal pain. Can that be enough to survive? Can living life in a world of trouble and pain with God by our side be enough? Can knowing one day there will be an eternity with no more tears, no more sorrow, and no more pain be enough to help us hang on?[32]

I have chosen to believe God is always listening even when it is quiet and still—even when the pain persists, the friend dies, or the cancer isn't healed. In the midst of my choice to believe that God's ear is turned to me, my choosing to believe God is listening turns to a "knowing." In the quiet and disappointment, amidst the incomprehensible and the grief, I surrender and remind myself of who I am and who God is. Despite the fact that He didn't save my friend's life, I remind myself that God is mighty to save.[33] Despite the lack of healing, I remind myself that God is a healer.[34] Despite my pain, I remind myself that God has faithfully loved and cared for me my whole life.[35] Though these unanswered prayers are at least disappointing and at their worst devastating, I remind myself that God promises satisfaction[36] and joy.[37] I try to remember and then just sit tight. Wait patiently. Hold on. Believe.

In time, I hear him again. I hear that whisper. There's a call to action. I see the wind blow. A shiver runs down my spine as the sun sets or the rainbow forms. I talk to someone who has understood for the first time God's amazing grace. I pick up the Bible and the words jump off the page and pierce my heart. A song of the redeemed is sung and I am completely undone.

In time—and usually quite a bit of it—I also see restoration. I see the brokenhearted dancing again. People healed. Ministries rising from the ashes of personal grief and devastation pouring out love on strangers who are suffering equal loss. In God's economy, within the restrictions of an imperfect world, he seems to be able to use *all things* for good. Even the most horrific. Eventually. If we let him and don't give up.

When I experience or witness any of that, the current answers to my prayers (or lack thereof) don't matter very much, and I just see Jesus. He is enough. Those moments and realities remind me that he is present and at work in our lives and in the world whether we hear him or not, whether we agree with his ways or not. When I take the long view, God's interaction, involvement, presence, and love are obvious.

Until.

In my distress I called upon the Lord; to my God I cried for help. From his temple he heard my voice, and my cry to him reached his ears.

Psalm 18:6, ESV

7

Heal Me. Trust Me.

Suffering marked her life… Nonetheless, regardless of her chronic and debilitating pain … still she came to the synagogue.

—Jo Kadlecek[38]

AFTER THREE YEARS OF DOCTORS APPOINTMENTS and an intense search to address my migraines, I found myself at a church in New Hampshire, surrounded by friends. My energetic quest "to get to the bottom of this" was a roller coaster ride. After each hopeful doctor visit or course of action, I was always left with the reality that it didn't work.

The morning sun streamed through the chapel windows, and my mind wandered as the preacher's deep voice played in the background. It felt good to be back in New Hampshire. Every summer since I was a toddler, I vacationed at this family camp on Spofford Lake. My memories here ran deep and wide. It's the place I learned to swim, water ski, play tennis, and sail. It's also where I had my first kiss, first boyfriend, and first best friend. Three generations of my life vacation here—my parents' friends who watched me grow up, former fellow campers and staff members, and now, my children's playmates. I can't think of a place I feel more relaxed, more known, or more at home.

Summer after summer, I sat inside these chapel walls, listening to stories about how God created the universe and Jesus made the blind man see, singing camp songs until my throat hurt, or laughing until my belly ached over skit night or some other silly presentation. Memories of campfires, tetherball games, the sweet smell of pine trees, 4th of July parades, kids singing, sitting in Adirondack chairs by the lake with family and friends—a million memories—collided in my mind. I was grateful for all of them and knew they were a gift.

Every summer I arrive at the lake hungry for a change of pace, new scenery, and a fresh perspective. This year was no different. I was exhausted by my headaches along with the weariness that comes with raising four children. Mike and I were eager to unwind and happy to have relaxation listed at number one on our "to-do lists." I desperately wanted this week to be light on the pain so I could enjoy time away with my family without the battle going on in the background.

I looked around the chapel and made note of who was there, anxious to catch up with summer friends. But as much as I tried to ignore it, the banging inside my memory laden head was distracting. I rubbed my neck, annoyed at pain's presence. Could I please get a break here? I tried to push it aside but couldn't. Earlier that day, I sat with my friend Debbie, complaining about this current migraine and recalled her suggestion to have the pastor who was speaking at camp for the week pray and "lay hands on me" for my healing.

Pretty bold idea, I thought.

I stared at Pastor Doug who was deep into his sermon (that I had yet to pay attention to) and wondered if he would pray for my healing. Was this a spiritual gift he possessed? Did he believe Jesus instantaneously healed people through prayer in this day and age? Did I?

I knew Pastor Doug from summers past and held him in high regard. He knew and liked this Jesus of ours with an intensity and intimacy that was contagious. His faith was real and passionate. His delivery of God's Word was always a unique blend of professionalism, excellence, truth, directness, authenticity, urgency, and love. I liked him. I also trusted him. Debbie's suggestion of gathering up some friends along with Pastor Doug to take some extended time and pray for my healing sounded somewhat appealing and yet terrifying.

I stared at him as he preached and wondered if I should. I had obviously prayed about my pain privately with God and asked him to heal me through the decades. Also, many others had prayed for me along the way. Why did this feel different? I think I was imagining those scenes on television with ministers laying hands on people in wheelchairs and they get up and walk. My friend Debbie was from a more charismatic faith background, and since it was her idea, I assumed she was planning on something a bit more "spirit-filled" than what I was used to experiencing in public. I have to be honest, some of those broadcasts make me uncomfortable. The prayer is noisy, and people are out of their seats. I was brought up in a more controlled church environment where no one raised their voice in church, put hands on a parishioner or got healed during a service. So, to ask the pastor and my friends to take the time to pray for my healing, together, at church, out loud—*to pray specifically and exclusively for God to actually heal me in real time*–wasn't a part of my spiritual experience, and it seemed a bit vulnerable and even weird. It also seemed selfish and demanding. My hurting head spun with reasons why I should have them pray for healing and reasons why I shouldn't. Why was this so hard? I needed to stop thinking about those healing services I'd seen on television and get a grip. Honestly, shouldn't we pray together to God, a God we believe to be loving and omnipotent, for healing? Issues of pride, doubt, protectiveness, and fear began building their walls.

Regardless of the mountain of thoughts filling my head and the resistance brigade making camp on my perimeter, I felt a push forward when the sermon ended—a propelling common sense telling me, "of course you and your friends should ask God to heal you." Yikes. I took a deep breath and decided I would humble myself and pray with Debbie, Pastor Doug, and any other willing friends present. Maybe. The service ended and I grabbed Debbie's arm to tell her what I was thinking. And before I could woo her into mulling over these thoughts with a nice, hot cup of coffee down by the lake watching the sailboats float by, she quickly replied that it was a great idea and ran off to get the preacher and our friends. (When it came to prayer, she was *very* enthusiastic.) Faster than I could say, "let's do this another day," we were gathered under the pine trees outside the church. I stood in the middle of my friends with Pastor Doug holding open his Bible.

First, Pastor Doug asked me a few questions about my headaches and then read some Bible verses from the book of John. The verses were encouraging. He read, "Whatever you ask in my name, this will I do, that the Father may be glorified in the Son. If you ask me anything in my name, I will do it."[39] I particularly liked the word "anything." "Anything" could definitely include my headaches. So, we placed our hands on the Bible and then they all placed their hands on my head and shoulders and started praying.

Before I really joined in mentally and spiritually with all the praying, I recall thinking how powerful the sense of touch was. How often do we lovingly place a hand on a friend's shoulder? I started to think about all those studies done in orphanages on the power of touch and how babies who were adequately fed but not physically touched would die. It felt strange, but incredibly kind to have their hands resting on me.

Focusing back on the situation at hand, I realized I had just jumped off a cliff into new territory. Since I was already in the free fall position, I opened my heart wide and engaged with God like never before (at least publicly)—asking for it all, for him to finally and completely take away this lifelong curse.

The preacher prayed for my head and claimed the promises of the Bible. As his words went up, I began to sense God's spirit coming down. I really wouldn't know what else to call it. The praying wasn't the sweet, orderly kind of corporate praying that I was used to doing. It was different. There was earnest, heartfelt longing, bold claims, and a groaning that came up from deep within me that was uninvited and uncontrollable. There were tears and more tears. There was frustration, honesty, amens, uh-huhs, and lots of "yes, Lords." My friend who never sheds a tear under the most moving of circumstances was bawling. I, like most people I know, wanted to be somewhat in control in this circumstance but definitely was not.

You know when you come to the end of yourself and whatever energy or adrenalin you've been using to get through is let go because either the difficulty ended or help arrived? While everyone prayed, I felt like that. I use a lot of my energy to counteract the pain in my head. In order to enjoy a day or someone's company during a headache, I have to work at staying engaged, not complaining, and getting the good out of a situation because the pain is always vying for my attention and focus. Although sometimes I have to succumb to the pain, mostly I try to fight it.

As I stood with friends, admitting my pain and helplessness before God with the hope that he might heal me, something inside me was released. I didn't have to "keep a stiff upper lip" and bear up under my burden at this moment. I was free to admit my pain and even hope for change. It made me weak in the knees. So, I held out my burden of pain and plainly asked God to take it away. Even though I had asked him before, there was something more empowering about doing it with witnesses with my hand on a Bible verse that told me that I should. Standing with friends who were agreeing with me as I asked made me hopeful. Listening to them ask on my behalf made me even more so. It was a completely pure and honest exchange. I was humbled as my friends stood in the middle of my pain with me, selflessly pleading with God on my behalf to heal me once and for all. I loved them for doing it and was overwhelmed being on the receiving end of such kindness.

As the preacher began to pray again, he paused and then prayed that I would have strength to endure the headaches if God chose *not* to take them away.

Did he say what I think he said?

Before he could continue, I stopped him. Who gave him permission to make *that* an option? I was claiming those verses we read and believing that the God who created the heavens and the earth could definitely take care of my little head. Why was he speaking of God saying "no." What in the world was he thinking?

"Pastor, I hate to stop all of this, but I have just as much faith to believe that God will heal me as those who were healed in the Bible, and I can't settle for anything less than that. Please, please don't pray that," I blurted out as I wished for a tissue.

I stared at him, and he said nothing. I assumed it was all cleared up, and I was ready to continue. I wiped my nose, bowed my head, and waited.

The preacher responded and I realized he wasn't praying. I slowly looked up.

"Eileen," he said, "maybe this is about trusting Him."

I wanted to throw up. He thinks I've had headaches for over thirty years so God can teach me about trusting him? Really? Was he serious?

"Trust me, it's not," I said.

I bowed my head again, wanting to continue praying for my healing. We were so close. It took me forever to get to this vulnerable spot and have others pray for me, to really pray for the miracle of healing. I truly believed that God would honor my obedience and heal me. I could practically feel it. I also figured God was anxious to heal me out of his love and pity for me. It was my time.

Trust? What did that have to do with it?

But he continued: "And maybe instead of bearing the headaches alone, you should let Jesus bear them with you. Eileen, I think you need to acknowledge Jesus in your pain and know he is *with you* bearing the headaches too."

I bent over and put my hands on my knees as if I just took a blow to the gut. I felt lightheaded as my feelings of hope started to evaporate while the preacher's words penetrated my mind. I didn't want Jesus to bear my headaches with me. I wanted him to take them away! The preacher's idea made me sick.

It's one thing to meditate on the truth that God is with us, but this was taking it a step further. To let God bear the pain also? To imagine God not just sitting with me while I am in pain, but to imagine him in pain with me–feeling what I am feeling, fighting what I am fighting. It intrigued me a bit, but since I was currently in the middle of asking God to actually heal me, I wanted to move on.

I have to admit that part of my sadness with these headaches is that the suffering is lonely. No matter how many caring people you have around you, when the pain comes, it is yours and yours alone. No one else can enter into it; no one else can take it for you. The pain begins and you have to be with it all by yourself. I hate that part. I have shared with my husband numerous times that I wish he could take on my head for a couple of days just so I could have his total empathy and know that someone gets it. If he could experience it just once, from that point on I could at least look in his eyes, in my pain, and know that he knows. It would help. I never thought of Jesus *knowing* my pain, experiencing it alongside me. The thought of him bearing my pain with me was jolting. For a second the idea made me feel less lonely and more loved. Perhaps if this healing prayer thing didn't work out, I would consider it.

The praying continued. It was like riding a wave, a crescendo and decrescendo, a cry and response until we all knew we were done. With a final "amen," we ended the conversation. I gave the preacher a hug and he left. My friends and I stood around for a moment taking it all in. It was mildly embarrassing. Someone summed it up with, "Wow that was something." No one dared ask the obvious question: Was my migraine gone? I suppose my silence communicated it wasn't. We just stared at each other for a moment until I turned from this precious group of friends and announced that I needed to go for a run. Luckily, I was dressed for one and off I went.

My mind raced as my feet moved. I needed to be alone and was glad when I turned the bend in the road and was out of sight from camp. The prayer, the Bible verse we read, my friends' voices and tears, the pastor and his idea, and the lack of healing filled me with emotion I didn't know what to do with—running was the perfect solution. There is something to that saying: "Go run it off." I was trying.

Over the next few miles, I spoke, pleaded, and continued to cry out to God. I wasn't done with him yet. I restated some of what we had prayed about and told him how much I wanted to "boast in the Lord" for his healing work in my life. I yearned to tell that story—the story of God's gracious healing after years of pain and suffering. I longed to be able to say that no one could figure it out, no one could give me relief, and no one could heal me except God.

I wondered how he could possibly deny me this. Wasn't it a good deal for both of us? It would obviously be great for me, and he would get all the praise and glory—along with some very positive publicity. I wouldn't be able to contain myself. I would shout out until the day I died how great God is, how powerful and gracious, full of mercy and healing power.

Still running, I wondered why I wasn't willing to shout that statement in my current condition. I believed in God. I knew he did great things. But I wasn't willing to shout his name from a mole hill, let alone a mountaintop. I suppose my love for God was full of conditions, disbelief, and ifs. If God healed me, I would shout his name. If God blessed me, I would serve him fully. If God proved himself to me in miraculous ways, this faith of mine would never waiver. If not, I'd just as soon keep him at arm's length, remain in charge, and let my doubts keep my life of faith in check.

My head screamed as my feet beat the pavement. And in the middle of my running frenzy, I realized that I was "a believer" who really didn't believe completely. Each time something didn't go my way or a prayer wasn't answered according to my request, I chalked it up to the probability that God wasn't all he was cracked up to be. I suppose I never *truly* believed God was in charge, ordering my days for a purpose and answering my prayers in his higher, and perhaps, better way. I was sobered by the fact that I believed all these truths about God with my head, but not my heart. After all these years of believing, I had to admit I wasn't very good at it.

On any given day, I would share with conviction that I believed God was sovereign and in control, his ways different than ours. I knew in my head that God knew more than I did and surrendering to his purposes despite our desires was the way to go. But when backed up against this wall of needing to let go of *my* desire for relief and surrender to his incomprehensible purposes, I couldn't do it. Instead of surrender and submission, my heart filled with doubt, disappointment, and resistance. At this crossroad, my theology was too hard to implement.

My legs were good, and I decided to make the left turn after the golf course and continue around the lake–about six miles. Sweat trickled down my back between my shoulder blades and my chest heaved. My head pounded along with my overworked heart as I rounded the bend, wishing for some water. I had already passed the tap of spring water that had been running here since I was a kid. No matter. I kept going. My tears mingled with sweat, and I turned my wet face upwards, looking past the pine trees to the blue sky and whimpered one more sentence to this God who was so perplexing and elusive, yet irresistible to me. Oh, he drove me nuts. Instead of a question, it felt like a conclusive statement. And I spit it out.

"You're not gonna heal me, are you?"

Silence.

I was coming up on my first hill and focused on climbing it. Nearing the top, I hoped I would hear him say he would certainly heal me, but I didn't. Instead, the thought that God didn't love me enough to heal my head taunted me. My heart sank. I assumed if he was going to, it would have happened in the moments Pastor Doug and my friends were praying—or at least by now. But my headache was getting worse with each mile I ran. I couldn't imagine why he wouldn't want to heal me and continued to land on the awful thought that he was lacking in love for me. I let this pitiful thought marinate in my soul for a couple of miles until I couldn't stand it any longer.

"He has to love me enough. You have to love me enough!" I spoke out loud as my stride got away from me coming down the hill.

It's everything I believe. It's what Christianity is all about. The fact that God loves us enough—plus more than we can comprehend—is the entire foundation of this religion, this relationship. If I threw *that* away, I might as well throw it all out and find some other movement, temple, or belief system. I huffed on down the road refusing to accept the awful idea of God lacking in love.

A holy resolve and some sort of righteous anger boiled in me. My body couldn't seem to contain the idea that God lacked love. And then, the thought shot out of my head like a cannonball. Something inside of me felt insulted by the concept and I let it fly away. With the horrible thought gone, I shook out my tired arms and hoped the feeling wouldn't linger. I kept running.

Hitting mile five, I figured it must be my problem, not God's lack of love. It must be me. It must be my lack of faith. That had to be it. The road rounded the bend, and I could see Spofford Lake clearly again. I loved how the scenery here looked the same as it did decades ago. When so much in life changes every year, the constants provide some glue. I took a deep breath and was surprised how bad my head felt and how strong my legs were.

I remembered as an eight-year-old kid sitting by this very lake one summer, wanting to test my faith. I had bought myself a necklace in the camp store with money my parents had given me. It was a small glass ball housing a mustard seed. The mustard seed was supposed to remind me of a Bible verse that says if you have faith the size of a mustard seed, you can move mountains.[40] I loved that verse because it made me think that God was kind and not so demanding. A mustard seed is miniscule and if that's all God required, I felt like I could be a part. How great that God didn't ask us to have a grown-up amount of faith, just a tiny, little bit of faith. It made me happy. So, I bought it, clasped it around my neck, and walked down to the beach.

I sat on a rock by the shore and proceeded to ask God to move the mountain. At eight, life was literal. I stared at the small mountain across the lake, holding onto my necklace, and asked him to move it over a little bit to the left—because I believed he could. I watched and waited, fixing my eyes on markers I had set on the horizon so I could be sure of when it moved and how much. I waited and waited, staring until my eyes burned. And waited some more. I sat there until the sun was about to set and the mosquitoes started biting. Slowly I gave up on the moment. The mountain never moved, and I left the beach feeling sad that my faith was smaller than a tiny mustard seed. I had thought it was so much more.

Envisioning the scene, I wished I could grab that eight-year-old girl and hold her tight in all her disappointment. I wished I could tell her that God couldn't move that mountain because if he did, people might die, roads would get torn away, houses would fall down, and all the life in that mountain would get disrupted, damaged and destroyed. Such an innocent request from a child who couldn't see or understand what God saw and knew.

I also thought about how God probably ached to answer her eight-year-old prayer, bolster her faith, and prove his reality and power—all the while knowing there was no way he could or would. As a parent, I related. My children occasionally ask me for something in their innocence and ignorance that I know I can't give them or do for them because it's not in their best interest. Even though it's hard for me to say no, I can say it with confidence because I—being older and wiser—know the ending. I know denying their request is the best thing I can do for them even though from their vantage point it's heartbreaking.

I imagine God feels similarly towards me as I feel towards my children. I want my kids to grow up into all they were meant to be, and I am usually not willing to exchange momentary satisfactions for long term results. I'm not going to say yes when I know—even though it may make them happy in the moment—it will not benefit them long term. I was also reminded that when I have to say no to my kids, I cannot wait for them to ask me for something where I can say yes. I wondered if God felt the same way.

Maybe I had enough faith, but just couldn't see or understand the reasons why God couldn't or wouldn't grant my request. Maybe.

I finally made it back to the beach and took off my running shoes. I was sweaty, and my legs were used up. Six miles were my maximum at that point, and I was glad to be done. Campers were starting to line up by the flagpole as the bell rang for lunch. I watched from the lake as I dipped my feet into the water. Just like they should be, the kids were wild—full of life, noisy, sweaty, hungry, and hysterical. The camp counselors tried to line them up for a quick mealtime prayer, and I watched as they bowed their heads. It made me smile.

My eight-year-old memory forced me to mull over a truth I knew but didn't want to apply to this situation: God asks us to have faith and believe even when we cannot understand what is happening around us. This is what faith is—believing in things unseen, believing even though it doesn't make sense—yet. I know this. But I wasn't asking him to do something that would hurt someone else. I wasn't asking for a materialistic desire or an intrinsic blessing. I wasn't even asking him to heal me from a year of migraines. I was asking for an end to over three decades of pain because I was worn out and desperate for relief.

It had been a long morning. Just getting to that healing prayer was a stretch for me—believing fully that God could do whatever it is we asked him to do and then letting my guard down—totally vulnerable and exposed before friends and God. Not an easy one for me. And now this—trusting God when his answer is no, trusting a God who gives and takes away. This trusting thing made the believing challenge look like nursery school. It was a whole other climb. A climb I didn't want to make.

I gathered up my sweaty socks and running shoes and left the beach. The kids were making their way into the dining hall, and the smell of fresh baked bread wafted through the courtyard—one of the many delights of camp life. I was hungry and thirsty, ready for lunch, and my head was still pounding. Well, if not today, maybe tomorrow, and, please, oh God, I am begging you—still allow the answer to this prayer be a resounding "yes." I couldn't think of a reason why moving this mountain would harm anyone and not be the greater good for me. I started back up to the camping area to shower, change, and wait for my healing. I said all I knew to say to God, and the ball was in his court.

My husband missed this particular morning at camp because he was out golfing with some other friends. As I walked across the campus, he caught up with me and asked about my morning. I just stared at him and smiled, too spent to rehash details. It would wait.

The afternoon was spent relaxing by the lake. I couldn't wait to sit in my beach chair and flip mindlessly through some magazine. Maybe I could spot on the ski boat while my girls went tubing. Or perhaps a canoe trip to the island to play on the rope swing. Matt and Cole would definitely want to do that again. But first, some water and a healthy portion of ibuprofen.

I awoke the next morning with a "top ten worst" migraine. Typical me, I thought. I finally get the 'healing prayer thing' done, and it makes me worse. I could barely lift my head off the pillow. During the night, I had woken up a couple of times headache-free and thought that maybe it was happening; maybe I would wake up with a wonderful story to tell and a happy ending; maybe God was saying yes. Mike, who had been brought up to speed on the previous day's events, looked at me with sadness and pity. I could barely speak when he asked how I was feeling.

Despite the nausea and banging, we made our way down to the chapel for the morning service. It was the last thing I wanted to do, but I was drawn nonetheless. Entering the chapel, I realized I couldn't go sit in my normal spot—up front—and we grabbed two seats along the rear wall. I plopped down, my head filled with searing pain, staring at the preacher who had prayed for me the day before. As he started preaching, I concluded that his spiritual gifts probably didn't include the gift of healing. I was distraught with disappointment and leaned into my chair wondering how the preacher's morning words would sound to my aching head and broken heart.

The negative thoughts and questions piled up: my lacking faith; the failed prayers; the ridiculous pain; the embarrassment; God's silence; God's no; the drilling in my face; cries left uncomforted; who is this God anyway? What kind of God wouldn't want to take pain away? Is this faith of mine real? What about that verse the preacher read? Did God have to make it worse? Are we all just making this stuff up?

And then a question interrupted my thoughts:

"Will you trust Me no matter what?"

What? I was spiraling down into my own personal pity party and along comes that trust thing again. The question hung in the air. It was loud and clear, inaudible and piercing. I looked around the room as if someone was playing a joke on me. I knew it wasn't *my* question or thought and slowly accepted it was God speaking to me—right there in my seat, in a crowded room, in the middle of a sermon, as if no one else was around. It was the one question I didn't want to hear and certainly didn't want to answer.

"Will you trust Me no matter what?"

I sat there, rubbing the bridge of my nose and temples trying to ignore him and hoping he would shut up. But he didn't, and I knew he wanted me to make a decision. Would I trust him? Mmm. Trick question? That would mean giving up my hope of one day being free of this pain, wouldn't it? No, I couldn't. That hope keeps me going. Why not heal me? Why did it matter to him if I trusted him to such a ridiculous degree? Wasn't the trust I had in God enough? Why was he being so demanding? I leaned forward and rested my head in my hands massaging it. I shouldn't have come to church.

"Will you trust Me no matter what?"

Enough already. I dug my fingertips deep into my scalp making circular motions all over my head. Mike leaned forward to check on me.

"Do you want to leave?" he whispered.

I shook my head no. The thought of getting up was too much.

"Your hair looks like a rat's nest," he smiled while rubbing my back.

I'm sure it did. I smoothed it over and leaned back into my chair. I sighed and rolled my head around trying to loosen up my rock-hard neck muscles. This was my second sermon with Pastor Doug this week and I still hadn't heard a word he said. I tried to tune in, but *that* question filled the atmosphere, and I knew I wasn't being let off the hook.

Will you trust Me no matter what?

Instead of struggling, why didn't I just give God a flat out "no?" Like, "No, I will not trust You." There. Done. Period. Over.

I considered it, but just couldn't do it. The thought of saying no to God made me feel like a fool. And, when it came down to it, I liked him too much. Who am I to think I know better than God Almighty anyway? Some clarity formed as I considered who I was and who he was. My grip loosened.

Would I trust him even if I never got to experience another week without headaches? Would I trust him if my headaches got worse? Would I trust that the God who made me knew what he was doing with my life? This battle was exhausting. For Pete's sake, if I can't trust God, who can I trust? Even though it was a lot to let go of, I put my head back in my hands.

I prayed again.

My eyes filled and I said yes. I would trust him no matter what happened—whether he healed me or not.

They were the most difficult words I had ever spoken, and if I wasn't in a crowded chapel, I would have sobbed. Then I picked up on Pastor Doug's suggestion from the day before. I asked if God would (please) share all of my pain with me, experience it, fight it, and suffer through it—an every minute, through the night, and into the next day type of companionship.

I swore I heard him say yes.

And in this supernatural moment, something swept over me. I'll call it resignation for lack of a better explanation. My fight to have it work out my way was over. I surrendered my desire for healing and prayed for the first time with complete abandon, "Thy will be done."

It's hard letting go of what you want—especially when it's been burning for a long time and seems like something you should actually have. But with the help of God, his Holy Spirit, and perhaps a host of angels working overtime, I was able to let go of my greatest, long-standing desire and accept whatever it was God was doing—or not doing. It had been a long wrestling match, but it was over. I wanted his way, no strings attached.

It was illogical. It was unexpected. It was reckless. It was crazy. Some would say it was dumb. And, when I think long and hard about that moment and what overtook me, I would have to say it was love—this unconditional, greater good, divine, victorious, complete, tough kind of love spilling out, pouring over, and covering my little world. It enabled me to do what I absolutely couldn't do on my own. It felt surprisingly great. And right. And true. And real. And complete. And it was over, along with Pastor Doug's sermon. Mike and I slipped out the back door.

Commit your way to the Lord; trust in him, and he will act.

Psalm 37:5, ESV

8

Show Me How to Live

The mystery of God's love is not that he takes our pains away, but that he first wants to share them with us. Out of this divine solidarity comes new life.

—Henri J. Nouwen

THE FOLLOWING DAY, I WOKE UP WITH A CLEAR HEAD and no trace of a headache. It made my heart race, and I was having a hard time controlling my excitement. The questions flooded my mind in a torrent. Did God bring me to yesterday to find out if I would trust him *in* my pain? Did I just pass some sort of spiritual test? Would he now give me the relief that I so desperately wanted? After a lifetime of living with headaches, was I finally done? Was this God's big surprise for me? A gift? A reward? I was too afraid to entertain the thought, too protective of my hopeful heart. If I started celebrating my relief, how much harder would it be to accept the next headache? I decided to keep it a secret until I was sure. This was an emotional rollercoaster ride.

How great would it be for my friends to see God answering our prayers? I knew how happy they would be for me and personally encouraged by the news. But the thought of telling them that the headaches were gone only to have to call the following week to announce a false alarm was too much for me. So, I didn't.

During the rest of that week, I woke up day after day pain free. It was such a relief having this break. Living without headaches is so much easier, and I was reminded of that truth yet again. I was happy to be enjoying a good run, especially since it was coinciding with our family vacation. I was practically giddy thinking it was maybe *more* than a good run; maybe I was healed.

When I am experiencing a string of pain free days, I am more fun to be with, more lighthearted. As Mike and I enjoyed camp together with the kids, I was reminded of that fact over and over again. Playing tennis without my head weighing a ton made it a whole new game, and running without something drilling into my face proved running more tolerable. My energy level grew after each pain free day as the absence of migraines enabled me to sleep. Aside from my enjoyment, I know my husband always finds "a pain-free me" more enjoyable—not to mention the children.

Part of my reason for not telling my friends and Pastor Doug that "God had healed me" was not only to protect me but God too. I have known a few people who were very ill and after much prayer seemed to be healed. The praises would go up, and then a few months later, the illness would reemerge. I really thought it made God look bad. Who wants to have a relationship with a God who seems to be capable of teasing? Sharing that God gives and takes away isn't very appealing. I certainly didn't want to be someone who turned people *away* from God. Wanting to spare God the bad press, I kept my mouth shut in case the headaches came back.

Which they did.

On day ten after we had returned home from New Hampshire, I woke up with my head full, heavy, and pounding. What in the world was going on inside my skull to cause this pressure, banging, and haphazard shooting pain? The fact that I hadn't felt any pain in more than a week made me see afresh how ridiculous and abnormal the activity in my cranium was. No one should have to live with this burden. I slowly got out of bed and told Mike my party was over. The pain was back. There was nothing to say.

I was relieved I kept the break to myself. I also took a moment to thank God for so many days of relief to fully enjoy my family and vacation. I couldn't overlook that blessing, despite my great disappointment. My sadness was tempered because of the caution I took. I half expected them to return, as much as I hoped it was over. When they did, it wasn't a big shock.

My decision to trust God whether the pain returned or not did spare me from going into a downward spiral. I had already let it all go at the chapel and amazingly felt a rush of freedom when the pain returned. I relinquished the reins and sat back in the saddle, curious to where God was taking me. All my unanswered questions could remain that way *if* I trusted him. I knew that was a big "if"—knowing myself as well as I do—but, I left New Hampshire resolved to do just that—*trust God no matter what*. I simply asked God if he would, day by day, show me how. Show me how to continue with the pain, how to take him with me, how to share the burden and do more than just endure.

I wanted him to show me how to live.

I heard a song blasting out of my son's room that grabbed my attention soon after returning from New Hampshire. The band's name was Audioslave, and their lyrics were surprisingly comprehensible between the screaming guitar and great beat of the percussion. I stopped at the bottom of our staircase listening in disbelief to the singer screaming my exact sentiment. When the song ended, I yelled upstairs to Matt, "Can you play that song again? And what band is this?" He shouted back, "Audioslave and the song is called 'Show Me How To Live!'" Okay now, you honestly cannot make this stuff up. No coincidence there. I scribbled down the lyrics as I listened again.

Encouragement and inspiration can show up in the most unlikely places. I don't really know what the songwriter, Chris Cornell, wanted to communicate with his lyrics, but, nonetheless, his words sailed out of my son's room, down the stairs and pierced my heart. I loved how he screamed out "show me how to live!" I asked Matt to crank the volume so I could sing along. Mr. Cornell sang with every fiber in his body how his Creator gave him the pain in his life and now needed to show him how to live. He and I were on the same page in word and level of urgency. Me and Audioslave. Go figure. When you get a chance, you should give the song a listen.

Settling into life back home, I was determined to implement my new revelation of "pain companionship" with Jesus that Pastor Doug had suggested. As the weeks progressed, my headaches were back ranging from intense and frequent to dull and occasional. I always get a few days break in between them, but they were continuing with depth and consistency. My belief that God acts in people's lives for good and for healing remained, but I, after this particular summer, realized more fully that eliminating our troubles wasn't necessarily his goal—and certainly not on his agenda when it came to me personally.

I was reminded of one of Jesus' promises—"in this world *you will* have trouble..."[41]—and was amazed at how I had glossed over and somehow ignored that biblical promise through the years. Hopeful I guess, but an act of denial for sure.

With "Show Me How To Live" playing in the background of my days, I was determined to find daily comfort and strength in Jesus. I was committed to trust Jesus no matter. I was also curious. If God wasn't going to heal me, I wanted to know what he was going to do. It had to be something. If he wasn't taking away my pain, what was his plan?

I needed a place to start, so I decided to begin each day, headache, and migraine by acknowledging God's presence and his desire to show me how to live. Simple enough, I thought. Every day I would lift my heavy, pounding head off my pillow, whisper a prayer for strength, and, once I dressed, got the kids fed, occupied, or—once September hit—off to school, I would land my aching body in the living room. There, I would open my Bible and begin my day by reading and praying.

I'm not the most disciplined person, but when desperate or wanting enough, I can sometimes override my nature and do something consistently, day in and day out. This was one of those times.

So, every morning I talked to Jesus about whatever was on my mind, asked him what he thought of the current headache, read some holy scriptures, and got on with my day.

After one particular morning session, I walked up to Grace's room where she was playing "house" to spy on her. She grabbed her dolls and fed them, played some peek-a-boo, and proceeded to lay them down for a nap. I watched her tuck them in with her cute, chubby hands and couldn't get over how adorable her green and pink bow looked against her shiny, straight hair. She then kissed their foreheads and took a seat in her miniature armchair sitting in the corner of her room. I wondered what she would do next and watched in earnest as she grabbed her little Bible and started "reading." At that moment, she spotted me.

"Hey, Gracie, what are you doing?" I asked, trying to sound like I just arrived at her door.

"Oh, I'm just doing what mothers do," she said in her little, matter-of-fact voice.

She looked back down at her Bible and kept "reading." I walked down the hallway with a smile, knowing my morning discipline was more apparent and consistent than even I realized. It was one of those good mothering moments when you get confirmation that your kids are not only picking up all your bad habits but your good ones too. I was grateful.

For the first couple of months of trying to include Jesus in my pain, my morning routine was accomplished by will power, mostly. But once September hit and Matt, Cole, Kit, and Gracie were in school, I found my routine taking more than twenty minutes. I thought maybe it was the luxury of time that allowed me to go slower, sit longer. But it was more than that. My conversations with God were growing into more than just reverently clipping through a list of thank-yous, concerns, requests, and an update on *our* (now that Jesus was sharing the headaches with me) pain.

In time, I found myself wanting to share more than the normal list. I wanted to expound on my thoughts, divulge my heart, whisper my dreams, and reveal a longing or two. Suddenly, I was confiding in him about a lost friendship, my pesky insecurity, or latest disappointment. I wondered what he thought of my current migraine and if the pain bothered him. Imagining Jesus massaging his head along with me while we persevered through another one was bonding. I likened it to trench warfare and the deep bond and sense of camaraderie that develops when two people live through a war together. A bit dramatic perhaps, but it worked for me. I not only spoke to God, but I also would just sit there and listen—believing he wanted a conversation, not a monologue, as much as I did.

We were becoming friends.

By the end of September, with my garden fading and Long Island's salt air turning colder, I started waking up earlier than normal, anticipating my time alone with God. Being that I am by no stretch of the imagination a "morning person," I found this phenomenon especially intriguing. Talking *with* God was so much better than praying to him. There was friendship in his presence, and his company was filling me up. As I spent more time reading the Bible and raising my awareness of his constant companionship, I couldn't get over how real he was—being invisible and all. Even though I believed in him and had prayed to him most of my life, this was different. It was more. It was better.

As the school year got underway, a women's faith retreat that I had been asked to help lead was looming in the distance. I decided I couldn't fulfill the obligation for a variety of reasons, but it was mostly because I had recently left the church—not church in general, just my childhood church in particular (sad story for another time). I told my sister and my friend Denise, whom I was supposed to drive up with, that I couldn't go, and they understood. Yet, as I contemplated how to tell the church's planning committee, I sensed God pulling at me to go despite my deep reluctance. I continued to pray, and, in the end, I knew God wanted me there.

Listening in faith for God's answers to my questions and opening up my heart, soul, and mind to his voice during the day was a better way to live. Despite the fact that God was invisible and inaudible, l was beginning to see and hear him. I must admit that acting on what I heard was a whole other step. No matter how much I believe in God's voice and what he is saying to me, it always requires a bit more to actually move on it. Let's face it, believing and acting on things unseen requires a true leap of old-fashioned faith. Maybe it gets easier with some practice. In the meantime, I pushed myself to listen and obey.

The retreat happened to be at Camp Spofford. Three months after my prayer for healing there, I was back in New Hampshire in the same chapel introducing the guest speaker who was about to begin her series on, of all things, "desperate women." If I had to choose one word to describe how you feel when living with pain, it would be "desperate." You are desperate because there's no controlling or escaping pain. You are at pain's mercy, and it has absolutely none. I thought God must have a sense of humor putting me back in this place with a banner of "Desperate Women" hanging over it.

I stared at our retreat teacher and wondered what inspired her to speak about desperation. You rarely teach on a topic that hasn't at some point had you as its pupil. I was emceeing the weekend and sharing the stage with her, so I hoped I would get to know her enough to find out. After making some announcements and delivering various thank-yous, I introduced Jo for the first time, and she made her way to the podium. She had a slight limp, and I wondered if it was a clue to what led her to this topic. I took my seat and knew I liked her before she finished her first five minutes. You can hear authenticity in someone's voice and see humility in their demeanor. Her eyes reflected the fact that she still found life funny despite the not-so-funny parts. Her words revealed a thoughtfulness and intelligence that made me want to listen. It was going to be a good weekend.

There was one Bible story Jo recounted that especially challenged me. It was about a woman who had been bleeding for twelve years, and no doctor was able to help her.[42] As a woman, it's awful enough to bleed once a month for a few days. Can you imagine hemorrhaging every day for years without a tampon in sight? Talk about miserable. In Biblical times, women were considered unclean during that time of the month and needed to remove themselves from their home to be with other women in the same situation.

Jo highlighted how this woman had to deal with more than her physical discomfort but also social shame and emotional pain. Learning of Jesus' visit to town, a man who could heal the sick and make the lame walk, sent her running to the streets to find him. After twelve years of exhausting all avenues for help, Jesus was her last hope. She believed he could heal her and made her way through the crowd until she got within arm's reach of his robe. She reached for it, hoping his healing power would flow out from him and onto her bleeding body. With one faith-filled touch, she was healed immediately. Her misery was over. As she trembled and testified before Jesus, her Healer, he commended her for her faith and told her to go in peace.

As Jo continued to unwrap this woman's story of desperation, faith, and healing, I became discouraged. Here I go again. Why her and not me? I had faith. I had reached out to this same Jesus, outside this very chapel, with the same hope of being healed. As I listened to the recounting of the story, it didn't matter that I had made a decision to trust God—healing or not. I realized it would always be hard to hear of others being healed while sitting in pain. I stopped my downward spiral as best I could, unable to stop the tears spilling out all over my knees.

After Jo was done teaching, everyone broke up into groups for discussion. I was obviously struggling with the story, and the gracious women in my group wanted to know why. I shared with them about my life with headaches and how I related to the woman in the Bible story. I told them how I believed as she did that God could heal, and, yet, he had *not* healed *me*. Even though I knew better, I couldn't shake that recurring, haunting thought that maybe he didn't love me enough or care. The awful whispers in my head told me once again my faith wasn't strong enough. Gosh, I know better.

I am beyond these lies. I wanted to silence it but couldn't. They were taunting me again. Despite my decision to trust God, I was still so disappointed.

Everyone in my small group knew me to some degree, but aside from my friend Denise and sister Betty-Ann, none of them knew I suffered chronic pain. They were surprised. (I was better at hiding it than I knew and more private than I realized.) As they passed me tissues to wipe my face, one by one, they started to share their pain. It was like my tears unlocked the door to everyone's hidden struggle, and within minutes, we were all talking about our secret pain—right there, in broad daylight.

But they also shared how despite their desperation, God also brought them joy. By the end of our heartfelt discussion, we were laughing through our tears calling ourselves "the cheerful women of pain." The juxtaposition of pain and joy was odd, but also relatable—joy, peace, and contentedness despite the suffering—I understood that. When we finished, I walked back up to the microphone to make some announcements regarding the afternoon and thanked Jo for making me weep. The meeting was over.

As I left the chapel, a few thoughts crossed my mind: first, we all have pain; second, if I hadn't shared my pain, the women in my group probably wouldn't have shared theirs. It's not that I am glad everyone has pain, it's just that I think if and when we do, it's probably better to share it. There's relief in the sharing and perhaps some healing. Lastly, I figured out the best way to render the lies (that taunt me) powerless was to talk about them immediately with some friends. If I let them fester in my mind, they could drag me into a struggle I didn't have to have. I walked out of the chapel with my head throbbing, but I was better, even so.

Throughout the retreat, God spoke to my heart like a certain scent speaks to your memory. He felt close and present. As strange as it sounds, I also felt his pleasure, and it kept making me smile. The weather was beautiful—a New England fall weekend that was warmer than it should've been. The sky reflected blue, the air smelled of leftover humidity and leaves, and the lake's voice hummed a peaceful tune as the summer boats and vacationers were long gone. I could hear myself think, and my heart rate slowed as life's running pace was replaced by a stroll.

Being away with Betty-Ann and Denise also refreshed me. It's not every day we get to take off the various hats we wear and put on the ones that don't get worn enough. Although I love being a wife and mother, it felt great to be a friend and sister. To be without my beloved entourage stirred parts of me that are usually shelved because of the work at hand. In between Jo's chapel talks, Saturday was spent chatting over coffee with friends, enjoying some beach volleyball, and then a canoe ride around the lake with some willing souls. For me, it doesn't get much better than that.

In addition, there was Jo. It's rare to meet a new friend who feels like home. As our paths crossed through the weekend, I could've sworn I knew her previously. I could tell she wanted to laugh as much as I did and cared about more than met the eye. She knew who she was and wanted to know more—more about anything—more about me, more about Jesus, more about the dinner menu. She was a relief and a surprise. I knew our introduction and the entire weekend was a gift from The One who wouldn't heal me. I had no idea how hungry I was for meaningful friendship. I suspected God did—which explained why I felt him urging me to attend this retreat. Those momentary realizations blanket my soul with a deep understanding that God cares for me in ways that are deep and wide.

In a conversation with my new friend, my lifelong battle with headaches came up. I'm not quite sure how since I rarely share these thoughts with perfect strangers. But there I was on the front lawn of the dining hall, chatting about my pain. I have to admit it felt good to talk about it and process out loud. Jo kept asking questions, and I kept answering them. She made me comfortable. She seemed interested. It was easy to open up.

Then the conversation turned to challenge.

"Hey, you should think about writing your story down," Jo plainly encouraged.

"Write it down? I don't think so," I answered, surprised at the idea. "What in the world do I have to say?"

"I think more than you know. Promise me you'll just try," Jo finished.

The thought of writing about my headaches seemed, to be honest, stupid. What was there to say? Who would care? Why would I write about my pain? My mind raced with the new idea, and I told Jo I would give it a go, fearful I was beginning this friendship with a lie. Even so, the thought resonated inside me and lingered long after our conversation. For much of my life, I had muzzled my voice, but in this moment, I felt a key turning in the lock that held it. It was subtle, but I was completely aware of the shift in my being. Maybe it was alright to speak up and out. Maybe I had something to say. The longer I thought about it, the more I realized there wasn't a soul on earth who shouldn't speak up, not a person who didn't have something to say. I would give it a try.

By Sunday afternoon, Betty Ann, Denise, and I were headed down the highway back to Long Island. Our conversation jumped from deep thoughts to favorite songs as the mountain scenery clipped past our windows. Our hearts were full with time well spent; our souls were satisfied; and our muscles were awake from the atypical extracurricular activities. In my bag was one of Jo's books[43] where I tucked her contact information. I was surprised she wanted to keep in touch but relieved by the invitation. After just a weekend of getting to know her, it would've been sad not to call her friend.

The weekend was a milestone for me, a point of culmination, an ending, and a beginning. I heard the sound of my voice and knew it was alright to use it, to speak out loud about the deep things and not worry about the cost of its release. I, for the first time, also thought my pain might have a purpose. It was already drawing me closer to Jesus and sharing it with others seemed to do some good for all of us. The possibility of purpose made the banging in my head feel more like a trumpet call than a death march, and it had hope written all over it for reasons I could feel but not understand.

The weekend also reminded me of how fortunate I was to have people in my life who have walked with me since forever ago. The common thread my sister and I share grounds me and offers a reference point that is unchanging. Denise, my friend since the fifth grade, knew me then and knows me now—keeping me honest about my life and continually reminding me of what unconditional love feels like. I felt rich beyond measure because of them. God's provision of a new friend in Jo also spoke of his love to me—his knowledge of who I was, where I was, and what I needed. He wasn't taking away my pain, but he was giving me what I needed to endure.

As the radio played, I let all these things settle into my bones. I thought of the various "desperate women stories" that Jo had shared, and it occurred to me that God's power wasn't just for those who were healed, but his power was also for me and anyone else reaching out in desperation. As much as I wished Jesus' healing power would cover my aching head, it wasn't happening. But just because I wasn't receiving God's *healing power* didn't mean I wasn't receiving his *power*. Maybe the power I received in reaching out was the power to endure. Not my first choice, but it was something.

The Bible tells many stories of the sick, blind, and deaf being healed by Jesus during his ministry on earth. I would venture to guess that there were many more people in his path that could have used a little healing and resurrecting, and yet he didn't heal everyone—even though he could have. It made me wonder again about his purposes, his goals, and his view on pain.

There's a story of Jesus encountering a paralytic that intrigues me. While Jesus was speaking to a large crowd gathered at someone's house, the paralytic's friends decide to bring him straight to Jesus to get healed.[44] They tried going through the front door to no avail and pushed back through the crowd and headed for the roof. Carrying their friend on a mat, they climbed up to the roof and started digging. Once they saw clear through the roof down to Jesus, they lowered their paralyzed friend on his mat and laid him as gently as they could at Jesus' feet. Talk about friends you want to keep.

When Jesus saw their faith (and I can only imagine his delight), he told the paralyzed man to "take heart, my son; your sins are forgiven."[45]

Take heart, son; your sins are forgiven?

I find Jesus' response to the paralyzed man—now at his feet—not only unexpected but strange. If I'm paralyzed lying on a mat waiting to be healed, I want to hear something more like "get up and walk!" I can imagine the expressions on the unhealed man's face and his friends—the anticipation, the confusion, and could there have been disappointment? Was the paralytic thinking like I was while reading this story? Sins forgiven is alright, but he came to be healed. He obviously wants to walk again!

I suppose we still don't get it.

If we're honest, most of us, when given the choice, want comfort, not holiness. I am afraid we don't fully understand the gift Jesus is holding out to us. I know I don't. In the end, Jesus heals the paralytic, not because he thinks the man is disappointed, but because the teachers of the law who were present accused him of blasphemy. "But that you may know that the Son of Man has authority on earth to forgive sins,"[46] Jesus healed the man and told him to go home. He healed the paralytic for *his* purpose. It seemed as far as Jesus was concerned, he had already given the paralytic everything he really needed. Sins forgiven.

I reluctantly concluded, again, that God's purpose is the soul of man, not our health or ease—which, in light of eternity, is a good thing. He knows that the healing of our bodies, the restoration of our comfort, and the easing of our pain won't necessarily turn our hearts to him. I don't know about you, but I usually look for a Savior when I'm in need of some saving. God knows our nature and maybe he allows our pain and suffering in order to draw us to himself, making us solely dependent on him for our next breath, to brave another day.

My pain is bigger than me. It makes me look outside of myself for help and forces me to turn my eyes upward. Consequently, knowing God and being in his presence becomes what makes my life better, regardless of my circumstance. Was this what the apostle Paul knew while sitting in a prison cell in chains, enabling him to sing in the dark?[47] Is this why the people of Haiti could gather at makeshift churches in the rubble and lift up songs of amazing grace after an earthquake devastated their country? Is this the phenomenon that causes great hope, unmitigated forgiveness, and songs to rise from the hearts of people who believe notwithstanding life's circumstances? How else can you explain a mother who forgives her son's murderer? Someone once told me a story about a young girl who wrote "Jesus Loves Me" on the wall of her brothel bedroom. Hard to imagine. God must be present in the middle of every mess, every darkness, delivering what's needed to the soul crying out for help. *He must be there.*

God's presence in the middle of our painful, messed up lives makes the difference. But here's the rub: I am often unable to receive the relief of his presence because my mind gets in the way—along with my pain, pride, skepticism, and lack of discipline. I also have to admit that more often than not, I *do* just want to be healed, not forgiven; comforted, not saved. Pain stinks, and I just want it to go away. I want to feel good so I can go about my business. I want to move on from all of this neediness so I can live my life the way I want to live my life. When my mind travels down that trail, it's crazy how hard believing and crying out become. And, without believing and crying out, God's presence goes unnoticed.

As much as I prefer a painless, trouble-free life, I don't know if I would find God there. I don't know that I would bother to look for him in blissful circumstances.

The women's retreat was one of those "mountain top" experiences for me. But, as always, staying on the mountaintop isn't an option. It's in the everyday grind that the truths I've learned and revelations I've received are put to the test. No matter how many times God blesses me with his presence or encourages me by his word, when the pain persists in the everyday, I have to battle to keep my ground and not fall back. I grit my teeth and remind myself of God's promises, love, hope, and purpose.

Sometimes I'm successful, sometimes not so much.

As my weekend retreat vanished in my rear-view mirror, I continued to start my days with Jesus, inviting him into my pain. I faithfully came to him, read his words, opened my heart wide in conversation, and listened for his still, small voice. Every day. My discipline slowly turned to desire and, without even noticing, showing up each morning to be with God became effortless. Alone with him in my living room was the place I longed for and anticipated daily.

I learned a few things that year. First, I do not suffer alone. None of us do. There are people right beside us who can relate and offer friendship. And, whether we know it or not, God is with us. Second, I discovered God was more conversational than I realized. Talking and listening in prayer was a better way to live, offering me relationship, not just faith. I was also beginning to realize that God was first and foremost interested in our holiness, not our comfort—which explained a lot. The realization that God offered his supernatural power to help us endure what was not taken from us began to crystallize. Lastly, it was sinking in that God cares about our pain and wants to bear it with us until the day he heals us altogether.

Pretty good lessons for a few short months.

Winter was coming to Long Island, and I felt the anticipation build with Thanksgiving and Christmas on the horizon—powerful days that offer love and a mysterious hope. I joined my kids in the countdown to holiday arrival, thankful for all the wonder around me. The brilliant autumn leaves fell, and the yard took on a sculptural presence. My front hallway started to fill up with snow boots, and the fireplace screens were covered again with drying socks and colorful winter hats while the kids, without fail or effort, made me laugh. They were quite the crew and a daily reminder of God's extravagant love and kindness towards me. My head continued to make me wince, and my morning habit sustained me.

I wondered what other lessons or truths waited for me in my living room. I knew there had to be more and was anxious to find out what they were.

Draw near to God, and he will draw near to you.

James 4:8a, ESV

9

Crazy, but True

I think all Christians would agree with me if I said that though Christianity seems at the first to be all about morality, all about duties and rules and guilt and virtue, yet it leads you on, out of all that, into something beyond.

—C.S. Lewis[48]

THE SEASON AFTER MY FAILED "HEALING PRAYER" with Pastor Doug and friends was riddled with an inordinate amount of migraines. My migraines and headaches were constant and were now lasting for weeks at a time. Some of the medications gave me relief, but, overall, the migraines were operating at a stronger, more persistent level. I couldn't remember a year when I felt much worse. Each bang in my head reminded me of Pastor Doug's instruction to bring Jesus with me into my pain. As a result, we continued spending an unusual amount of time together. Really unusual. I practiced this new "technique" until it was automatic. I couldn't forget Jesus during my day in the midst of my busyness because I had associated him with my pain to such a degree that they were synonymous. Since my pain was chronic, Jesus was now chronic.

Before, my response to a migraine or "headache run" certainly wasn't spending an inordinate amount of time praying, reading, and singing myself through the pain. More often than not, I would brace myself, try to ignore its existence, or use distractions to get my mind off it. But now, my pain was a call to quietness, a call to Jesus—my direct line. Was this how God wanted me to live?

The more headaches I had, the more time I spent with him. Sometimes I wondered if God was manipulating me with my pain. Since my pain called me to him, did he allow the constant stream of headaches just to be with me? If he did, I forgave him since our time together offered relief and company. The more time I spent with him, the more I liked him. As the days and weeks progressed, my pain and God's presence were one, and I found myself more able to endure my discomfort because he spiritually sustained me. It sounds nuts, but how do you explain a relationship with God?

The New Year came and went; the winter vacation ended, sending the kids back to school, and my daily pain dropped me to my knees praying for God's presence and strength. My headaches had elevated and elongated to such a degree that my normal routines were being affected. It was turning out to be an incredibly bad year. Although I am well practiced at the art of "carrying on," I have my limits. I pulled myself from tennis, stopped going to the gym, limited my contact with friends, and scaled back on family activities and engagements—which left me alone to cope. It was basically just me and Jesus.

The days would pass something like this. Matt, Cole, and Kit got the first school bus in the morning. We were fortunate enough to have the bus stop right at the end of our driveway, allowing me to wait on our front porch with the kids until they ran off. The porch overlooked our front lawn that was shaded by two 100-hundred-year-old Norway spruces. Our fence ran along the road until it opened up at our driveway gate. When the weather was nice, the kids would play out front, shoot hoops in the driveway, play on the swing set, or sit with me while I sipped my coffee, talking about their day ahead. As the bus pulled to a halt, I would wave watching as my incredible kids, Matt, Cole and Kit, ran to catch the bus, shouting their good-byes and jumping on with their backpacks bouncing behind them. Grace's bus came soon after the older kids', and once her little legs climbed on board, she waved to me through the window. Gosh, I could eat her up. After blowing kisses her way, I would go back inside to meet with God Almighty—who was waiting for me in my living room.

Rounding the corner of the front foyer, I creaked my way across the old pine floors and landed on the couch. My Bible lay waiting on the coffee table. The piano stood ready for a song, and the bay window next to the fireplace framed the view of our side yard—which consisted of more spruce trees regularly filled with an abnormal number of red cardinals. I knew God was present and waiting. A great way to start a day.

My head hurt most mornings, and I would begin with that, but the most amazing result of my new method of coping was that I quickly moved on—anxious to share God's company, read the Bible, sing him a song, or listen to his thoughts. The pain was secondary. I was drawing close to God, and he, as promised, was drawing close to me.

Sometimes I would read part of a book from an author who seemed well acquainted with him. Sometimes I would pray for a few minutes. Sometimes I would pray for hours. I would sit and listen with my heart and feel led to read some more or pray for something or someone more specifically. Sometimes I would wander over to the piano and fill our time with songs about how great he was and how much I loved him, or I would play an old church hymn where the lyrics suddenly made abundant sense. Sometimes, I would listen to his "voice" and hear, "Get off your knees and get to work." Those moments made me laugh and realize God not only wants our company but appreciates the fact that there are things that need to get done.

As my time with God grew, so did my desire for more. I don't really know how to describe it outside of a thirst or hunger. I knew there was infinitely more of him to enjoy and know. There was a big difference in my relationship with God compared to previous years—the greatest being that now my desire was not for what he could give me or relieve me of, but, rather, my desire was just for him. There were no longer strings of healing attached. He was no longer a means to an end, my wish granter. I just wanted him.

There was joy in his presence. It was interesting being with him. Our time together ranged from philosophical meanderings to contemplative repentance, worship and praise, to doubt and questions, from satisfaction to feelings of homesickness. He was intriguing, funny, smart, gracious, understanding, sympathetic, loving, and ridiculously kind. I wasn't surprised by my findings. I had studied the attributes of God but just never experienced them to this extent.

Another delightful finding from our time together was that he liked me—a lot. Since I was a young girl, I knew that God loved me—and every other person on the planet—I just hadn't realized how much he liked me. It felt better than love and I could feel my head lift and shoulders pull back knowing I was cherished, valued, and enjoyed by, well, God. Humility and pride co-mingled with the thought, leaving me covered by an overriding sense of security and contentment.

By the end of February, my desire for God hit an all-time high. I decided I needed Jesus to visit me. Ideally, I wanted him to knock on my front door, sit at my table, have lunch, and stay for a long visit. I wanted to see him face to face. I wanted it more than I ever wanted anything—knowing full well that God doesn't physically show up in our age, knowing I needed to wait until eternity's arrival for such an experience. But, I wanted it anyway.

My time with God, aside from being both enjoyable and satisfying, was also building my faith. Even though I chose to believe in God at an early age, I rarely experienced him. There were moments but never a daily awareness of his presence. But now, I couldn't deny his presence, and it was making my faith stronger. I knew it was impossible to spend hours in my house alone praying, reading, singing, and talking to someone if there wasn't someone there. But, there was. My experience and relationship with God were added proof of his existence. As the saying goes, "it takes two to tango," and I certainly was interacting with someone.

The more I acknowledged God's presence, the more my desire for him grew. It was a strong, constant nagging that resembled the longing of love and yet it was bigger, broader, deeper, and higher. It was bound to happen after spending so much time with him. This feeling lingered day after day and followed me around like a new puppy constantly sniffing at my ankles and scratching at my door. It had that Christmas morning anticipation that simultaneously collided with the reality that Christmas was over and wouldn't be returning for another year. I was beginning to feel homesick right in my own living room knowing that I wanted more of God but having no clue how to get it. What do you do with an invisible God when you want to see him face to face?

The longing for Christ continued with reminders of him that started popping up everywhere. It was a beautiful moment. A song. A Christ-like person. A glimpse into his character, his grace. It was the breeze, that sunset—that ridiculous over-the-top sunset when the sunbeams stream out from behind the pinkish, purplish clouds. I saw God in my kid's crooked, crazy smile. I heard him in the music. In a beautiful voice. I saw him in my garden, at Costco, on the athletic field. Everywhere I was, he was. Always trying to whisper something in my ear. The longing for more of his presence would surge when I bumped into someone who seemed to know the same God I knew, and I would want to do a 180 and ask if they'd like to find some others and live communally 'til the end of time singing songs around a roaring campfire. It really was getting ridiculous.

Can we have more of him? Are we able? Are we allowed? Or, are we placed here, purposely designed not to be able to get too comfortable so we keep looking heavenward straining our eyes and ears to catch another glimpse?

Sometimes even the not so spiritual helped quench my thirst. For me, the presence of God is often strong at an event involving lots of people. I am not sure why. Maybe it's all those souls in one place. Maybe God likes special events and celebrations. Perhaps it's the music and the aesthetic of the environment reminding me that "every good gift and every perfect gift is from above, coming down from the Father of lights."[49] Whatever it is, a good party with some interesting people works for me. The conversations are stimulating; I dress up, eat good food, drink fine wine, and maybe even dance to a live band. It makes me happy and thankful. A night like that can satisfy my yearning to a degree and remind me that Jesus is not only in my living room, at church, in the sunset, or in my pain, but (thankfully) at the party too. I love that about him. But each time I hung my dress back up in the closet, I realized my yearning for more of him was still there.

I couldn't figure out a way to quench my thirst for more of God and frustration was building.

I decided to try a new approach. Perhaps if I limited my time with God, I wouldn't want him so much and my frustration would wane. (A bit counterproductive, but I was desperate.) I laughed at my "all or nothing" approach and how I now felt the need to limit my interaction with him if I couldn't have it all. It was during this time that I began to understand Saint Paul's statement, "For to me to live is Christ, and to die is gain."[50] I never understood or wanted to believe that verse. Who wants to die and leave their friends and family? Who wants to give up on life and all its potential? Even though there were many days when I thought anything would be welcome if it took away my pain, I never wanted to leave the tangible and dive into the unknown—even if it did mean relief from the suffering. But now, being more acquainted with this Christ whom Paul spoke of, I knew that death *would* be gain. If he could deliver such peace and joy in the midst of my life on earth how unbelievable would it be to live in his physical presence with the promise of a new body and the absence of everything bad?

So, I started to water down my contact. A few nice readings from Proverbs. Not too much music. Prayers filled with requests and needs instead of the heartfelt, authentic dialogue that brought me too close, wanting more. But even with my concentrated effort to withdraw, my longing for him persisted, and I was driven to do something, anything to calm it or make it disappear.

So I got as busy as my head would allow.

A project seemed a helpful diversion. My daughter's room looked rather bland, and I decided to paint a mural of the English countryside, which would take weeks. After that project, I addressed the kids' longing for a pet. Being that we lived on what was once a small farm, I thought chickens would be fun and practical with the bonus of fresh eggs. So, I did some research and prepared our yard for chickens. Aside from the new projects, I allowed myself to get swept up in the normal busyness of family life, and my morning routine with God was curtailed. After the kids went off to school, I no longer started my day with him in the living room. Instead, I limited my contact to a quick prayer here and there. As I backed away from God, he let me go. I don't think God is one who elbows his way into our lives. He comes where he's wanted.

The focus of my day was caring for the kids, house, meals, friends, extended family, and various commitments. There was plenty to distract me from God, and I think I might have forgotten about him if it weren't for my pain. My headaches wouldn't allow me to wander too far. When the banging inside your head hurts enough to stop you, what else can you do but cry out to Jesus. Aside from needing him, I have to admit, I missed him too.

Sometime in May of that year I went back to starting the day with him in my living room. After just one extended morning in prayer, I was reconnected and felt the pleasure of his company. He didn't waste a second.

As the days passed, that nagging feeling for more of God returned. Geez. I couldn't stand not having it all and so refused to give up on my idea of a house visit, lunch, and a look at his face. My stubbornness was evident, and the desire was strong. I wanted to see him face to face just like Moses.[51]

One morning I stumbled across a passage that resonated with me:

> For we know that the whole creation has been groaning together in the pains of childbirth until now. And not only the creation, but we ourselves, who have the

> firstfruits of the Spirit, groan inwardly as we wait eagerly for our adoption as sons, the redemption of our bodies. For in this hope we were saved.[52]

I concluded that we are supposed to "groan inwardly as we wait eagerly." How could we not? If we have a taste and have caught glimpses of God, how could we not be left waiting for his return? The groaning reference struck a chord in me, and I was reminded that along with the groaning there is, thank goodness, all that hope—a hope I can almost see and faintly hear. I closed my Bible and rested it on the coffee table with some understanding and peace but also disappointment in the waiting part. I don't want to wait. I can barely wait for my computer to boot up without getting agitated. Forget about waiting until eternity for more of him. But what could I do? I decided to resign myself to the limitations of faith—disappointed, yet happy to be back to my routine of mornings with God.

On the last Friday in May of that year, Mike and I planned on going to a church service with some friends. They had invited us a couple of weeks earlier for an evening of music and worship. My friend and kids' piano teacher was playing with the orchestra, and his wife was singing in the gospel choir. I looked forward to a night of such singular focus.

My family attended a small Presbyterian church, so when I walked into my friends' church that Friday, I was impressed at the size of their sanctuary. There was a large balcony over the auditorium where cushioned seats offered a comfortable spot to relax and feed your soul. The stage was filled with musicians—a full orchestra, huge choir, drums, guitars, electric pianos, and my friend at the grand piano. I tried catching his attention before finding my seat but couldn't and sat down. Slowly the auditorium filled, and the chaos of musical noise formed a chord as the minister made his way to the podium.

He was a handsome, Italian looking fellow dressed in a suit and tie. He opened by explaining how we had all been invited to God's house for the evening. He used a metaphor of how he and his wife anticipated a friend's invitation for dinner, and when arriving at their home, they eagerly stood at the door and knocked. The hosts, obviously home, invited them in for an evening of fellowship and eventually a meal. He continued to say how we were in God's house, and he is home waiting for you to knock on his door so he can invite you inside to fellowship with him. As he spoke, every nerve in me awoke. This sounded like my persistent desire. How did the preacher know?

I decided my desire for God to knock on *my* door and visit with me at home could surely be reversed. I could come to *his* house instead. It seemed a fair trade. I whispered a prayer to Jesus telling him that I could certainly come to his house and thanked him for inviting me. With that, I smiled, thinking the whole night was for me, and the choir burst into song, filling every square inch of the building with voices and instruments beautifully shouting: "I will praise you in the sanctuary! Yes, I will!" I closed my eyes and whispered "yes, I will" a few times before joining in the song. Glory be.

Have you ever been in a church service where you thought someone had told the preacher all about you and your particular dilemma? This was one of those nights for me. The worship and music continued, and I drank down both, feeling what I had been longing for...satisfaction. I was amazed at how God graciously brought me to this particular place on this particular night to answer my aching heart with his presence in the midst of this music and sanctuary. It was perfect.

As the worship and music continued, I was reminded of my desire to also see his face and have lunch with him. I wondered how he would accomplish it. In between the various songs, the gentleman leading all the musicians kept repeating one phrase: "The presence of your face." He said it as the music played behind him and repeated it over again. I stared at him confused. What in the world does *that* mean? Why did he keep repeating the phrase? Clueless, I closed my eyes and concentrated on the words: "presence of your face." I still couldn't figure it out. I just tried to picture God's face—not knowing what else to do.

I conjured up a strong image filled with wisdom and time along with piercing, kind eyes and a slight, but wonderful, knowing smile. I threw some shine around it, since he is God, and just enjoyed the moment with my made-up Jesus face. After the interlude, the choir kept going and led us in a song with lyrics inviting us an into God's sanctuary. As the sopranos soared and the lower voices came behind them, grounding everything with some beautiful harmonies, the lyrics implored us to come, to come and stand face to face with God. The orchestra was on fire, and my friend was pounding the keys while the lyrics repeated the invitation to come and stand face to face with God. Bingo. At that moment, I knew God was saying, "That's the best I can do for you right now with the face thing." It was more than enough. God's attentiveness to my desires both humbled me and made me want to laugh out loud.

At the end of the service, the pastor led the congregation in prayer and asked if anyone wanted to pray with someone for healing in their life. Along with the many, I went up to the front to find someone to pray for my chronic headaches and migraines. Although I had obviously already tried the healing prayer thing to no avail, I figured it couldn't hurt to ask again. (You should never give up on the possibility.) My current migraine was on day twenty-three and I was tired and desperate—as usual. I saw all the designated prayer people with long lines in front of them and was struck by the evidence of a hurting world. I couldn't understand why the Italian looking pastor stood alone on the stage and I decided to approach him. I climbed the steps and tapped him on the shoulder.

"Pastor, would you mind praying for my chronic migraines?" I asked, feeling slightly awkward.

He looked confused and I suddenly realized he was facilitating the evening and not planning on praying for individuals, so he could pay attention to the room as a whole. The couple of dozen folks on the floor of the sanctuary were assigned the task of praying for the many who had come up for healing—not him. Before he could say a word, I apologized.

"I'm sorry I didn't realize you weren't praying. The lines were just so long, and you looked free. I am so sorry," I said as I started backing away.

He grabbed my arm and suggested I go pray with his wife who was standing stage left with a long line in front of her.

"Great idea. I'll go do that. So sorry," I mumbled, turning to go down the steps.

He grabbed my arm again. I think he felt badly for me. He put down his microphone on the floor and said,

"Here, let me pray for you. What is your name?" he said smiling.

"Eileen and I have had chronic headaches since I was a young girl," I blurted out.

Before he prayed for my head, he put his hands on my shoulders and stared me in the eyes and said—ever so slowly,

"Eileen, this is your meal."

Are you kidding me? I was paralyzed by his words knowing he had no idea about my crazy "lunch with God" yearning. It felt like a direct hit. I tried to focus as he prayed for my headaches (which seemed quite secondary at that moment), and when he was done, I quickly slid back into my seat. I was dumbfounded by God's desire and willingness, and perhaps even his sense of humor, to answer my longings with such clarity and kindness in a single night.

At the end of months of longing for Christ—for him to come to my house, to see him face to face, to have lunch with him—my desires were satisfied. There I was in his house, staring at my made-up face, and being told by the pastor that I had received my meal. I appreciated God's efforts to answer my prayers and it made me feel known by him, seen and heard by God the Father. It was a good night.

I realize this all might seem crazy, stupid, or even insignificant. I get that. But, when you really think about it, shouldn't our spiritual lives look, sound, and feel different from our physical lives? Shouldn't there be another dimension when it comes to relating to God? Hasn't there always been? Don't we all have to be a little crazy to join with the angels singing, hear an inaudible voice from God loud and clear, and have everyday happenings supernaturally take on great meaning, command all of our attention, and even turn our lives around and upside down?

What encourages me greatly—when I feel especially "out there"—is that I am not alone. For centuries, people have decided to follow God and live spiritual lives of devotion that have caused them to hunger, thirst, and long for more. People like the Apostles, Martin Luther, St. Augustine, Abraham Lincoln, C.S Lewis, professional athletes, authors, artists, politicians, family members, neighbors—an endless list of people from the past and present whom I admire for their ability to believe in things unseen.

I rest knowing there's a diversity of folks who testify similarly regarding this personal God. Our common denominator, Jesus, has made himself well known to many—people from different cultures, socioeconomic backgrounds, and personal experiences. It amazes me, and I am convinced again of God's universal appeal and both his ability and desire to get to know any and all of us—whether it's because we are crazy enough, desperate enough, smart enough, simple enough, honest enough, humble enough, or lucky enough to let him in.

Sometimes I think I let God into my life to the extent that I have because I am crazy, but then I reject that notion because, well, I'm not. Sometimes I know it's because of my desperation. Other times, I'm sure it's because of my intelligence—until I recall those SAT scores. Then there are days when I believe it's my simplicity, honesty, and humility—even though I'm not very simple, honest, or humble. Most often, I think I am just lucky that God tapped me on the shoulder and got my attention. Lucky enough to feel his affection and know his love. Lucky to have a God who wants me to know who he is, to know what he's like, to know what he thinks.

Yeah, basically I think it's "luck."

The natural person does not accept the things of the Spirit of God, for they are folly to him, and he is not able to understand them because they are spiritually discerned.

I Corinthians 2:14, ESV

10

More Doctors…

I know they meant to be just as good and kind as possible. And when people mean to be good to you, you don't mind very much when they're not quite—always.

—*Anne of Green Gables* by L.M. Montgomery

DESPITE THE LESSONS I WAS LEARNING, the physical and mental toll of my pain demanded more doctor appointments. That's the thing with chronic pain: you make progress in dealing with it, you answer some of the questions it stirs up, but as time passes and pain persists, you cannot help but circle back around, finding yourself at ground zero again some days. Pain is hard to live with, and you can never get perfectly comfortable or resolve it to the point of absolute peace. At least I can't. Pain nags and you must keep contending with it—revisiting the questions and rediscovering the answers. You also have to keep looking for help. Something that will alleviate the pain. Something that might cure it. You have to keep trying.

I decided to go back to one of my general practitioners who had treated my migraines when I was in my mid-twenties. I had lost touch with her when we moved out of state, and even though she never found a solution for my pain, I recalled her thoroughness, professionalism, and desire to help me.

Come appointment day, I walked into her office and was immediately transported back in time. Nothing had changed, which I took as a bad sign. The décor, smell of the office (distinct, but not unpleasant), and the ugly prints framed in gold metal that flanked the worn-out waiting room couch were exactly the same. She greeted me with the kind face I remembered, although I couldn't believe how much older she looked. I am sure she was having similar thoughts about me.

Dr. Rider had miraculously hung on to my records and asked about the effectiveness of the medicines she had long ago prescribed. I had tried a few prescription drugs with her, none of which worked long term. I wasn't the best patient back then and had never given her feedback or follow-up. But, I was finally telling her that the last prescription drug she had given me worked for quite a while but then seemed to lose its positive effect on me. After that final try, I had really just given up on prescription drugs, assuming they weren't for me. Despite my frustration, I was grateful for the consolation prize of being *painfully* drug-free—aside from my over-the-counter pills of course. (Believe me, if any of them *had* worked, I would have committed myself to prescription drugs for the rest of my life and been grateful. But since they didn't, I claimed the obvious benefit.)

Dr. Rider was surprised I hadn't found a solution over the years, but she also knew how elusive migraines and headaches could be. She looked sad, and I welcomed her sympathy. I tire of keeping that upper lip stiff and sometimes just want to take a break and wallow in self-pity. So, I sat on her table and moaned for a bit while she nodded and took some notes. She encouraged me with the fact that the medical community had made progress in the pain department, and she had a prescription in mind that had been quite successful in treating migraines. I was ready to *not* be drug-free and eager for relief. After a full battery of blood work and a general check-up, I took her prescription and drove away from the outdated office, excited to swallow something that promised to knock my pain from here to California.

The next day I woke up with a migraine and drove to the neighborhood drug store to fill the prescription on my way to a charity luncheon being held at a friend's house. The shop was crowded, and I politely made my way to the counter and handed over my slip of paper. I noticed the shelves filled from floor to ceiling with bottles of pills and syrups and was struck by the enormous role drugs obviously play in our lives. This pharmacy was one of many in town. How many pills does it take to carry a neighborhood of people through the week? The thought overwhelmed me as I scanned the shelves loaded with bottles and paper bags. Yet, I was more than ready to join the ranks and was genuinely excited when the pharmacist called my name. I paid, asked for a glass of water and popped the pill before getting in my car.

Let the magic begin.

It wasn't long into the drive that I started to feel my hands tingle. I had no idea what to expect and was thrilled that my body seemed to be reacting to something. Perhaps the tingling that had started in my fingers would continue up to my head and give my throbbing skull relief. I came to a stop sign, which I absentmindedly rolled through and soon after heard a siren and saw the red blinking lights in my rear-view mirror. Ugh! I pulled over, slowly came to a complete stop and waited for the police officer. Upon his arrival at my open window, I immediately confessed my sin—apologizing for my laziness in not stopping. He asked me where I was headed and I told him, thankful it was a charitable event.

The good officer, surprisingly and graciously, let me go with just a warning. Before I drove off he looked into my eyes and said in a low, husky voice, "Don't be in such a rush." Good advice, I quickly thought. As I continued, it seemed everything was obeying the police officer. The world seemed to be moving in slow motion, and, suddenly, it was impossible for me to drive faster than a moped.

The tingling had reached my head.

I meandered into the house filled with women enjoying each other's company. The smell of chicken, fresh salads, cakes, and cookies hung in the air. I kissed friends hello and made my way through the chatter to the kitchen counter and grabbed the only empty seat. My entire body was fuzzy and felt as if I had drunk a couple of glasses of wine too many. I helped myself to the food, thinking I had better start eating. My body's reaction was accelerating, and I was getting nervous. I quickly began shoving food in my mouth (which wasn't necessarily suitable for the occasion) fearing I was about to pass out. I thought the more bread and salad I had in my stomach, the better chance my body had of absorbing the drug, causing the negative reaction to stop, or at least slow down for Pete's sake!

I turned to a friend sitting next to me as I faded away.

"Danielle," I said, grabbing her arm for support, "I just took a new migraine medication and I think I'm having a bad reaction."

Her eyes opened wide as she exclaimed, "You're white as a ghost!" She helped me to the couch.

Danielle immediately took charge and rallied others to join her. Lying down, I was grateful to be horizontal in the living room and not crumpled in a heap under the kitchen counter. I deliriously mumbled that the medicine was in my bag and then surrendered myself to their care.

With the room spinning, women's voices whispering, and nervousness in the air, I started to think about the rest of the afternoon. Within the hour I was supposed to show up at my daughter Kit's classroom to help them make Valentine's Day cards for a local nursing home. We had also planned to surprise the kids by coming in with special cards made for our own child. Kit's card was at home.

I grabbed another friend, Dawn, and spoke about my dilemma. Without hesitation, she called the school to inform the teacher of the situation and got someone to take my place. Then on the coffee table next to me, she started making a card for Kit. Ah, friendship. Then, I felt my throat tighten. I told Danielle, who was frantically reading the paperwork accompanying the medicine, to call the doctor. She told me I seemed to be experiencing all the negative side effects that were listed and I should probably go to the hospital.

Why I didn't listen to their good advice is beyond me. In my delirium I thought the situation was dramatic enough and being rushed to the hospital seemed overwhelming. I told them I would go if the symptoms worsened and closed my eyes, praying to God they wouldn't. My friends acquiesced, though I have come to believe that you should probably never defer to the decision-making of a drugged person who cannot even stand up. Fortunately, my symptoms leveled off, and I fell asleep.

I woke up when I heard Dawn leaving for my daughter's school with the newly made card and noticed my dear, nervous friend Danielle still studying the pharmacist's notes. Others were trying to contact my doctor, and I slipped away again, bewildered as to what happened between my body and the pill. Closing my eyes, I was grateful to be surrounded by such good women.

I awoke to my cloudy mind and Dawn's face offering me a ride home. I was able to finally get off the couch and crawl into her car. The party was over and so was any possibility of this drug's usefulness. I was thankful when I arrived home that I had some time to rest before the children got off the bus. I curled up on our couch and dozed off again.

A few concerned friends called to see how I was doing, along with an old acquaintance who must've wondered why I sounded so groggy in the middle of the afternoon. The latter called to ask if I would be interested in leading a prayer group to pray for the schools in our district. Exhibiting amazing self-control, I stopped myself from laughing and without explanation or hesitation, told her it wasn't a good time for me to lead a prayer initiative—which probably confused her more. When is it not a good time to pray? All I could think about was how I could barely get myself through the day, let alone support a school district by leading a prayer team. I hoped she'd find someone more suitable.

Dr. Rider finally called and told me not to take any more of the pills (as if I would) and suggested I go see a neurologist. She gave me Dr. Blank's number and a glowing recommendation. I must admit she seemed hasty in pushing me on to the next doctor. I guess she figured she tried twice to help me to no avail. I made my next appointment with the neurologist and went back to sleep.

As my husband and I drove back to retrieve my abandoned vehicle that evening, I was well enough to worry about what all the women at that lunch thought of me. I felt ridiculous on some level, but too tired to give it real time and energy. I was curious to see what the next doctor would do with me. Frustration crept in, and I fought to remain focused on a solution.

The following week, I walked into the neurologist, Dr. Blank's office—which was sobering. There were wall to wall people, some in wheelchairs, some with walkers, and others with obvious neurological problems which, honestly, made me uncomfortable. I looked like a picture of health and younger than all his patients by at least twenty years. Do only the elderly have neurological problems? Would I end up in a wheelchair? I took a seat and completed the paperwork.

The wait was surprisingly short considering the volume of patients. Dr. Blank didn't work alone. I walked in and shook his hand, encouraged by the kindness in his eyes even though he looked tired. His desk was piled high with papers, and he appeared overbooked like most physicians these days. His face was harried. I believe he was someone who would've cared if he had the time. I felt sorry for him. We went through my history and discussed my recent adverse reaction. He proceeded to prescribe another migraine medicine that had been quite successful in relieving my kind of pain. He said he was putting me on the mildest dose due to last week's episode and told me to call him in two weeks to review my progress. I was encouraged by his confidence.

I left his office hopeful the medication would be better than the last one and began taking it the following day. As I neared the end of my two weeks, I (along with the rest of my family) noticed I wasn't quite myself. Despite my pain, I have usually been able to remain true to my personality, which is more upbeat and energetic than sad and lethargic. By week two I was, simply put, depressed.

I have had periods of sadness in my life caused by death, hard times, tragedy, or a series of really bad choices, but I've never been sad for no apparent reason. It was awful, and I felt imprisoned by the heaviness. My sadness quickly coupled with apathy, and within days, I apparently didn't care about anything or anyone. As I shrugged off my children and sat emotionless at the kitchen table, I realized the new medication was not only taking away my pain, but life as I knew it. Alarmed, I jumped in my car and drove to the doctor's office to register my complaint.

It wasn't until I arrived that I realized there's no doctor in the metropolitan New York area who would ever see a patient without an appointment. I don't know what possessed me to drive over and drop in without a phone call, but there I was. One of the administrative assistants arose from a sea of desks and telephones and walked toward the counter where I was standing. She gently asked me how she could help. I told her I needed to see the doctor immediately, but for just a couple of minutes.

She, of course, explained that I needed an appointment, or he could possibly call me at the end of the day. I blurted out that the medicine Dr. Blank had prescribed was making me very depressed and my entire personality had shifted. Without delay she turned to go get the doctor. From across the room, the kind lady nervously shouted for me to "please take a seat and give her a minute!" Wow. I was stunned by the immediate service and concern.

Within a minute (or maybe less), the doctor was at the counter speaking to me. He pulled me to a quiet corner of the waiting room and asked how I felt. I described my current lackluster state and how I didn't care about my family anymore. I told him it was really hard to get up in the morning and start the day because I seemed to be void of desire and adrenalin. I went on about how what used to make me laugh seemed moronic. Then, in the midst of apologizing for my awful personality, he grabbed my arm and said,

"Eileen, I have to tell you that the two possible side effects of this medication, albeit remote, are depression and schizophrenia."

Well, that certainly explained the last couple of weeks. You think maybe they could've warned me.

Looking concerned, Dr. Blank continued, "Please throw away the remaining pills immediately after you get home. I am so sorry for this side effect, but please know I prescribed the mildest dose."

His concern was mingled with defensiveness even though I wasn't blaming him for anything. I just stared at him and nodded.

"Okay then, Eileen, do you think you can drive yourself home?" Dr. Blank questioned, looking apprehensive.

"Well, of course, I can. I drove myself here," I responded, wondering if he knew something I didn't. Did depression impair my ability to get behind the wheel and steer myself home? Should I call a taxi service?

He grabbed my elbow and took a good, hard look at me. I returned the look and said, "Yes, Dr. Blank, I can get myself home."

"Alright then, let's get you an appointment for tomorrow morning," he said, leading me to the receptionist who was waiting at the counter.

I made the appointment and wandered to the elevator in a gray fog. Dr. Blank followed me.

I tried to smile and told him I would see him in the morning. The elevator doors shut, and I stared at the slit between them until they opened on the ground floor. I slid into my car and looked forward to throwing out the bottle of pills when I returned home. Give me a migraine any day. Being pain free is not worth sacrificing feelings of contentment, desire, and hope. Anger, irritability, and frustration even seemed welcome compared to this current void. Depression is a funny thing.

The next day I dragged myself out of bed, sadly shoved my kids out the door for school, and returned to the neurologist's office. Dr. Blank decided migraine medicine wasn't going to work for me. The two medications I had taken over the past month were "proven winners" and had been prescribed at their mildest doses. He was concerned that I would continue having extreme adverse reactions to anything prescribed and believed we needed to approach my head from another angle. First, he wanted an MRI of my brain and scheduled me for the following week. I said good-bye and walked through the crowded waiting room again. I passed the many neurologically impaired patients and wondered what was at the end of this road for me. Amazingly enough, in the state I was in, I didn't care where I landed. I shrugged away my thoughts. Nothing seemed to matter.

As the medication left my system, it was as if the clouds parted on my heart, soul, and mind. I relaxed again without wondering about the meaning of life. My energy and desire to help my kids with their homework returned. Doing chores wasn't like climbing Mt. Everest. A day was once again something to be enjoyed, not survived. Being depressed is horrible, and I realized what a gift contentment is, even when coupled with pain. No one should have to slog through days like that.

I added those who suffer with depression to my prayer list, and my headaches, once again, seemed a blessing in comparison. This earthly existence is not easy, and for some it is a living hell. Believing in heaven as I do, I wished God would come quickly and establish that place the Bible talks about where there are no more tears and suffering.[53] Talk about hope. In the meantime, thankfulness for my pain grew, knowing it was better to feel something than nothing at all.

When I returned for my MRI, I was relieved to learn that my "scan" was going to be done with an "open MRI." Normally, you are put in an enclosed tube for the photo session. An open MRI is just that, open on all sides allowing exposure to the outside world all around. I observed the round table on which I would lie, and the large circular disk of about the same size suspended above it. Being that I am mildly claustrophobic, I was deeply relieved not to be shoved in a tube that certainly would have caused panic on my part.

The nurse interrupted my thoughts and asked me to go change into a hospital gown and wait for the technician who would come and escort me back to the MRI room. I followed her instructions and marched into the dressing room, feeling more nervous about the scary possibilities than I was willing to admit. The technician soon arrived and knocked on my dressing room door. I cautiously opened the door, stuck out my hand and formally introduced myself.

"My name is Roger," he said, returning the introduction with a smile that out matched mine by a mile. "Let me show you around the place!"

Roger was young and noticeably enthusiastic about his job. His black curly hair was full and shiny. His eyes apparently weren't as healthy as his hair. His glasses were thick, and he was having some trouble keeping them on the bridge of his nose. I figured he must be in his twenties. His accent confirmed he was born and raised in the New York area. I let go of his hand. When I am nervous, my mind races, and I have to try and occupy it. Gathering first impressions about the person in front of me helps distract me from my nerves and keeps me in the moment—preventing my mind from racing off to all the possibilities and things I can't control. I get weird in doctors' offices.

Roger asked me again if I wanted a tour of the place, and I snapped out of it. He showed me his booth where he would be imaging my brain and then the adjoining room with the ominous machine where I would be for the process. He continued to try and engage me in conversation, which slowly turned to a ping pong match of light, personal questions. I clutched at my robe as I participated in this cocktail conversation—finding it hard to ignore that I was here for a brain scan, not a social engagement. To Roger's credit, his friendliness won me over and soon I was relaxed enough to return the chatter.

We stood at the entrance to the MRI room, which was dark with blue, glowing lights. Roger pointed out the various pieces of equipment, and I listened like a good student. The machinery was sleek and modern, giving the impression of a movie set for a science fiction thriller. He showed me where I would be lying and how the apparatus over my body would lower down to take pictures of my brain. The atmosphere was as soothing as a place like this could be with the blue lights, and I felt calm and ready until I saw the helmet.

The helmet was affixed to the table, and I was expected to put my head in it to assure I wouldn't move during the MRI. No one had mentioned this part. Roger assured me it would be fine and told me to slide my aching head up into the helmet. I obeyed. He then pulled the cage down over my face and secured it. (Have you seen the movie *Silence of the Lambs?)* Now tell me, what good is an open MRI if your head is locked in a helmet blocking any view of the outside world? I may as well have been in a tube. When the large, heavy, saucer-like contraption lowered, hovering inches above my body, I was no longer comfortable. Unfortunately, I started to panic.

Roger had left the room and was now speaking to me via a microphone from his control center. I was able to communicate with him through the sound system and quickly explained that I was a bit claustrophobic and felt trapped. Roger told me he could pipe in some music to help calm me down. His voice was perky, and he seemed pleased with the thought that he could remedy my situation with such ease. I was thrilled at the suggestion and asked if he could find some James Taylor.

Within seconds JT's acoustic guitar and sweet voice filled the room. I love James Taylor—always have, always will—and Roger was now my hero. I thanked him profusely as we engaged in some more light conversation and had a few laughs. Seeing I was calmer, Roger excused himself from the conversation to begin his work. I, with confidence, told him to go about his business as I hummed away my every fear. As he took pictures and did whatever else he had to do in his computer booth, I decided to do some leg calisthenics to the rhythm of the music to pass the time and distract myself more fully from the fact that I was screwed to a table and pinned between two large, heavy flying saucer-like disks getting a brain scan.

Right before the leg calisthenics, I started to reminisce about my spelunking days out in South Dakota during college one summer when I was trapped in miner's clothing with a flashlight strapped to my head in a crawl space measuring twelve by twenty-four inches. A group of us from a geology class were crawling through a tiny tunnel thousands of feet under the earth in an effort to get to an underground cave of stalagmites. I thought I would die down there as fear and claustrophobia set in. My friends literally had to drag me through as I hyper-ventilated. The leg exercises in the MRI were my attempt to ward off the bad memory and avoid comparing it to my current situation.

After a few minutes, Roger was on the loudspeaker again, this time sounding somewhat exasperated. He asked what I was doing and explained that even though my head was secured, the leg exercises were jostling the machine and obscuring the images. He told me to lie perfectly still as he now had to start over. I apologized and tried to explain how I was doing it just to keep calm, but he cut me off and repeated that I needed to lie still. Knowing Roger was upset, I did my best to be as still as a rock and focus on James Taylor, not spelunking.

Roger kept telling me how much longer I had left in the session, which was helpful, and right when my ability to ignore my confinement was waning, he announced we were done! I was so excited that I had remained calm through the process that when Roger said I was done, I impulsively wrenched open the helmet, pulled my head out, and started shimmying my body out from between the saucers.

I froze when I heard Roger yelling at me over the intercom. "What are you doing? Stop! Who said you could get yourself out?!"

I laid there frozen until he came into the room with my legs dangling out of the machine while the rest of my body remained sandwiched between the saucers. I couldn't believe how upset he was. I yelled to him from beneath the saucer,

"Roger, I've never had an MRI before and had no idea I wasn't allowed to take the helmet off and get myself off the table. I'm sorry! I was just so relieved it was over. You didn't tell me I had to wait for you to take me out..."

"Don't move. Stop talking and just wait for me," he yelled back.

Ugh.

He raised the large disk above me, enabling me to finally sit up. Roger went over to take a closer look at the helmet. His voice was loud and upset again as he exclaimed, "You broke the helmet! Do you know this costs $40,000?!"

I tried to calm him down. I pleaded my ignorance, apologized for the helmet and assured him the helmet couldn't possibly cost $40,000. I was certain the entire machine did, but I didn't break the entire machine! The helmet couldn't be more than a couple of hundred dollars. I told him I'd pay for the damage. I was sorry. He was such a nice guy. He played JT for me. I couldn't believe how mad he was. He told me to "just leave the room." So, I did.

Once dressed, I came back to his booth and apologized again.

"Roger, I am terribly sorry," I said, waiting for a response.

He wasn't interested.

"So," I continued, "how does my brain look?"

Without making any eye contact with me, he said, "I can't say. The doctor will go over the results with you at your next appointment."

I felt bad for Roger, knowing I had probably gotten him into some sort of trouble. How in the world did I break that thing? I wondered if they really would charge me for the damage and what my husband would say. Did insurance cover situations like this? Would it cost $40,000? Would my children go to college?

My only solace was that Roger was angry with me. I figured if he had seen a tumor inside my brain, he would've felt badly for me and not been so ticked off. I was almost sure I'd get a good report from the doctor at my next visit.

I returned to the office within days, thankful Roger's area was separate from the neurologist's office. I flipped through magazines, waiting for them to call my name and wondered what the doctor knew about the broken helmet and my visit for the MRI. I prayed Roger wouldn't walk in and see me. I kept the magazine high and my head low just in case. I decided if Dr. Blank didn't bring it up, I wasn't going to mention it. I hoped Roger resolved everything without involving the tired doctor.

Once they called my name, I made my way to the examining room, climbed up on the table, and waited for the doctor. He came into the room smiling and announced that he was pleased with my brain images which were clear, showing all was healthy. I knew it.

With all that good news and no mention of the broken helmet, I asked him what we were going to try next. He told me he was sending me to his colleague who was going to discuss a muscular treatment. Oh. Just when I thought he was gaining a slight understanding of my condition, he passed me off to yet another doctor. I walked down the hall to the new office and waited on yet another examining table for the next doctor.

He walked in and greeted me with a long stare. He resembled Albert Einstein with his wild gray hair and mustache. I hoped he was as smart. I answered some of his headache questions and pointed to the areas of my skull that were normally affected. In the middle of my description, he interrupted me and assured me he wasn't "making a pass," but he felt compelled to compliment me on my appearance. Excuse me?! I stared at him, speechless. He reassured me of his professionalism and asked if I would just accept his compliment. What's a girl to do?

I suddenly felt self-conscious and humiliated. Having "Dr. Einstein" focus on my outward appearance made me think he didn't care so much about my inward dilemma. How unprofessional could he be? I was mortified. I was also worried that his preoccupation with my outer layer would distract him from my three plus decades-long problem of pain.

I imagined telling the doctor how inappropriate it was to compliment a patient on her physical appearance, how he should be ashamed of himself and beg my apology. Unfortunately, all I could muster was a pathetic "thank you." Thank you? I'd been too surprised to be nimble on my feet and come back at him with a well-deserved tongue lashing. As strong as I think I can be at times, I often disappoint myself with my wimpy responses. I just sat there—wide-eyed—muttering "thank you." Not a proud moment for women's liberation. Gosh, going to the doctor shouldn't be this hard.

Then he told me he wanted to inject my neck, head, and face with Botox to calm what appeared to be overly excitable nerve endings which could be causing my migraines. He explained how this treatment had worked for about fifty percent of his patients. I asked a few obvious questions. I knew people used Botox to make their wrinkles go away. The injections paralyze your muscles, making your face relaxed and wrinkle-free. I think it's a form of botulism. I worried I wouldn't be able to squint my eyes or furrow my brow. Would I be able to hold my neck up if he was to paralyze those muscles too? He assured me I would function fine, and it was worth a try. He had to order the Botox and would call me to set up an appointment when it came in.

Along with the Botox injections, he suggested regular massage with therapists trained in pain management. I couldn't believe my ears. At the end of this journey, Botox and massage were the answers? Really? If relaxing my muscles were the answer to my problem, I felt lucky. There were so many other possibilities and outcomes I had contemplated while visiting the neurologist's office.

Nevertheless, I was afraid of Botox. I was sure that I would be one of those people whose eyes would droop after the injections, and I would never be able to smile fully again. The massage therapy just seemed too good to be true. I left the doctor's office knowing I felt too self-conscious to walk back into his office in the near future. But, I would put these simple ideas on the back burner and consider them for sure.

That was the end of another school year and another round of attempts to get rid of my headaches. On my drive home, I said a prayer listing a hundred things I was grateful for—first and foremost, a healthy brain. No matter the trouble, there is always something incredible that fills my heart with gratitude. I whispered a prayer of thanks for the good brain scan and no mention of the broken helmet.

This past year I had felt God's company in a way I never had before—because of my pain—and now wondered if I was afraid to let the pain go. Would I remember Jesus in my days if I actually had no more pain with which to contend? Was I putting off the possible solution of Botox and massage therapy because now, in a strange way, I didn't want my pain to disappear—fearing Jesus would disappear with it?

I remembered the story of Jesus healing a lame man at a pool called Bethesda. Jesus is walking by the pool and sees the lame man lying there and has compassion on him. He approaches him and asks, "Do you want to be healed?"[54] I've always wondered why he would ask a lame man if he wanted to be healed. Today was the first time I didn't think it was such a dumb question.

Summer was approaching and my kids would soon be with me 24/7, leaving no more time for doctor's appointments and complicated thoughts. For now, I decided to simply look forward to days at the beach, my routine of pain, and the glorious distraction of July, August, and children. Pain relief would wait. My headaches would be around come September, and I would resume my pursuit then.

I pulled into the driveway and admired the red roses dangling over the white fence. The baskets of purple verbena hanging on the front porch were overflowing which made me smile—along with the sunflower seeds Kit and Grace helped me plant that were now two feet tall. The grass was thick and green, and my dog Beau had his face plastered up against the bay window in the kitchen, waiting for me. I smiled again, put my car in park, and went inside to greet Beau and get ready for my kids, who would soon be dropped off at the end of the driveway by the big yellow bus. Life was good, despite the pain.

> *Not only that, but we rejoice in our sufferings, knowing that suffering produces endurance, and endurance produces character, and character produces hope, and hope does not put us to shame, because God's love has been poured into our hearts through the Holy Spirit who has been given to us.*
>
> Romans 5:3-5, ESV

11

A New Song

Come Thou Fount of every blessing, tune my heart to sing Thy grace; Streams of mercy, never ceasing, call for songs of loudest praise.

—Robert Robinson

THROUGHOUT THE SUMMER AND THE FOLLOWING YEAR, God's pull on me continued to be magnetic. No matter what was going on, I couldn't start the day without him. My pain served as my reminder, and my time with him reading, talking, listening, and singing proved to be not only helpful but a whole host of adjectives from delightful to sustaining. Outside of my living room, our communion was constant, and I included him in all my waking hours. He was such good company and never seemed to tire of me or my aching head. Then, something new happened.

I was sitting in church one Sunday—bored—and started jotting some thoughts down on a piece of paper. I wrote them in a verse and chorus format, and as I approached the chorus, I began to cry. I'll never forget it. The sun broke through the stained-glass window, and I could feel it heat up the top of my head. I believed it was the presence of God. I went home, sat at the piano, and put the lyrics to music. Within a few minutes, my thoughts were a song. I wondered what made me think I could even write a song in the first place. I never had before.

The past year of drawing closer to Jesus worked both ways; he was drawing closer to me.[55] His presence was palpable, and, as a result, I found myself looking for ways to respond to him. I suppose music was a natural outlet since I always appreciated its draw, depth, beauty, and ability to transcend the moment and add the subtlety of meaning that unaccompanied words often lack. Music makes me hear differently. It allows words to be louder and clearer. It ushers them past my mind right into the depths of my heart. I guess that's why it's been called "the language of the soul." Quite perfect really. When words and actions are not enough, music takes me places I need to go.

A couple of years earlier I could never have written a song. It was only through eavesdropping on my children's piano lessons and the gracious mini lessons received from their teacher that I learned anything about chords and progressions. Surprisingly, I now somehow knew enough to sit down and put my thoughts and emotions to music. It wasn't necessarily good music, but enough music to allow me to express my heart and work out my faith in another way.

After my first song, I went on a roll. When driving, a song would occasionally form in my head, and I'd quickly call my voicemail to sing it over the line so I wouldn't forget it. The songs would come all at once—within minutes I had both melody and lyrics. There were times when I would sense one coming and sit at the piano and wait for it, like a meal was about to be served. Almost suddenly, there it was—words, melody, verses, chorus, and even the occasional bridge. If I got stuck on a phrase, I'd wait a second for the words to finalize and scribble them down as fast as I could while tears dropped onto the piano keys—because I knew it was from God.

I know it sounds strange, but that's how it was.

When I had written over a dozen songs, I started believing that I was a songwriter. God, knowing my love for music, had been gracious enough to help me find a way to connect with him in this new dimension. I thought it was fantastic, not to mention utterly enjoyable. A song would come about twice a month or sometimes twice a week, and I began to wonder what to do with all this music until, suddenly, it stopped.

It was strange to me when a couple of weeks had passed, and I hadn't written anything new. I decided to go sit at the keys to get the juices flowing and conjure something up. Isn't that what songwriters do? Sometimes I had a good reflection or revelation from the day, and I thought, *Heck, now that I'm a songwriter, I can just write a song about that*. But, alas, I would try and try, and nothing would come. I couldn't write a song if my life depended on it.

For me, it seemed that my songs bubbled up as a direct result of keeping company with Jesus. They didn't come from me, but him. I couldn't write anything that made musical sense on my own, a fact made clear time and again when I tried to will a song into existence—as well intentioned as it was. My music happened when God inspired me, not when I tried to inspire myself. In the unexplainable, sweet communion between God and me, something good happened.

The good part wasn't just the joy of inspiration and creating something new, but my head felt better when I sat at the piano. Sometimes the pain would even disappear while singing. I wondered if singing moved and relaxed some of my muscles which allowed the pain to stop. Other times, the pain didn't stop, but I was focused enough on the moment that I didn't feel the pain in the same way until the singing was over. Both of those possibilities made me sit at the piano and sing more than I probably would have without them. It was helpful.

Along with that observation, I also realized I wasn't a songwriter, but, instead, a good listener and—I say this with due humility and awe—a friend of God's. I wondered what else I would hear besides songs if I continued to tune my ears to God's voice. I recalled moments when I had "listened" to God's prompting and did something good when I didn't have the time, possess the courage, or have the inclination. Promptings to make a meal for someone, complete a mundane task for a family member, tell someone how much God adored them, or even write a book. In hindsight, I knew it was God's soft whisper that pushed me to do what was better—though inconvenient and, occasionally, even nerve wracking—for the simple purpose of love. Those moments—when I listen—always leave me feeling full, satisfied, part of something bigger than my little life, and I wonder why I don't listen more often than I do.

I accepted the fact that God enjoyed my company and gave me songs to sing. At this point in my life, the music served a few purposes. First, the songs were heartfelt worship that enabled me to sit for hours and sing to God my praise and adoration. (Don't knock it until you've tried it.) As items on my "to do" list went unchecked, I sat alone with him in my living room and sang what was in my heart. Aside from the worship, the songs strengthened my faith. The lyrics I wrote down spoke truth. The fact that something dynamic, tangible, and beyond me was happening helped me believe more. I felt his power and love through the music, and it drew me closer. Lastly, the songs provided a way for me to work out my faith. Along with my questions and doubt-filled lyrics came God's words of truth, affirming my faith, encouraging me to believe again, and convincing me of what was, what is, and always will be.

One day as I was vacuuming up dust bunnies, rotating loads of laundry, and swirling cleaner around porcelain bowls, I began to wonder what it would be like if I truly believed it all. What if I believed the whole thing from the Garden of Eden[56] to the Promised Land[57]—from the manger in Bethlehem[58] to the cross with the nails, the soldiers, and the thief?[59] What if I believed every last word of the story from the transfiguration[60] to the empty tomb[61]—from Christ's ascension[62] to the day the Holy Ghost blew through that upper room with a loud, rushing wind and tongues of fire?[63] What if I believed the promises—from joy unspeakable[64] and all surpassing peace,[65] to a love that never fails?[66] What if.

Sooner rather than later, I found myself at the piano, exchanging my duster for a pencil, scribbling down my question filled verses.

> What if I believe the God of all creation came to earth
> because He loved me?
> And what if I believe that the One who drew the heavens had a plan for you and me?
> What if I believed…What if I believed…
>
> What if I believed that the God of all glory knew my
> thoughts and deeds?
> And what if I believed that He loved me still and
> longed to meet my needs?
> What if I believed…What if I believed…

But the chorus felt more like a declaration and revelation as those questions sunk into my consciousness, and I realized:

I'd sing Glory Hallelujah! What a Savior! I would praise His name forever. He's redeemed me! What if I believed? What if I believed? What if I believed?

After a few more verses and a bridge, the song wound its way to a final phrase repeating "yes, I believe" for as long as I felt like singing it. Every time I sing that song, I feel my faith build and my heart inexplicably fill up with a soaking sweetness—which I suspect is joy. I don't know about you, but it is hard to come to God. Singing often moves me beyond my doubt to confirmation where I know there is nothing and no one truer than him. When God's grip on me is tighter than my husband's, I am able to believe in things unseen with surety. It's in that place that I feel joy unspeakable and experience a love that never fails—and everything around me makes a little more sense.

Along with the songs, I was also writing about my pain. On a flight to Chicago for a college reunion, I decided to keep that promise I made to Jo at the women's retreat to write about the ever present pain in my head. With a blank journal resting on my little snack tray 30,000 feet up in the air, I picked up my pen and started. When the flight attendant announced we were arriving at O'Hare, I laughed, thinking how time really does fly and wished I was on a flight to Tokyo so I could keep filling the blank pages with a million thoughts, opinions, and questions regarding this pain of mine. Who knew I had so much to say? Perhaps if I got it all out of my head onto paper there'd be some sort of pressure release and the pain would stop. You never know.

After months of writing, Jo shared some of my headache story with an editor she knew. He was interested, and after I submitted an abridged version of some of my writing, he wanted to publish it in a magazine. The thought of letting perfect strangers into my world was nauseating, but I figured if my words were helpful in any way to someone in a similar situation, it would be worth enduring the vulnerability and dread. So, I said yes.

After the article was published, Ed, the editor (no joke), was kind enough to forward some of the readers' responses. It was a gift to hear from fellow sufferers and compassionate souls. I was deeply moved by their faith and courage. The thought that my pain brought anyone hope or encouragement was simultaneously humbling and worthy of celebration. To have your pain be worth something to someone—if only for a moment—adds purpose to the suffering and changes the entire situation—in a good way.

Many of the emails directed to me were filled with well-intentioned advice. Most I appreciated while some, I must admit, just plain annoyed me. Some suggested remedies I had already tried. Others offered completely novel ideas I had never heard of for treating head pain. Who knew that some people found relief by avoiding "night-shade foods"? What *are* "night-shade foods," and who knew they existed? Some advised me that if I eliminated the stress in my life, I would find relief. I thought of Job's friends from the Old Testament. Others suggested a variety of drugs. I even had one person tell me that she had been fitted with a purple-tinted pair of glasses to correct her perception and sensitivity to light patterns. She was totally healed from her migraines. Hmmm... Would my vanity allow me to try *that* solution? Not so sure.

Then there were the emails that offered no advice. I remember reading one from a 17-year-old girl from Kazakhstan who had suffered mild headaches every day for the past few years, which had just progressed to migraines. She shared how the doctors told her they were hereditary and how her mother also suffers from them. "Hereditary or not," she wrote, "that doesn't relieve the pain." I empathized with her as she described how she was "climbing the walls" because of her migraines and felt like God was far away from her. But then she wrote that after reading my article "she realized it wasn't God who was hiding from her, but rather she was hiding from God." She went on to thank me for helping her realize that "even with my headaches God is with me and loves me, and that I should love Him and trust Him too even if the pain doesn't go away." Wise beyond her years. If I knew where Kazakhstan was, I would have jumped on a flight to go see that 17-year-old girl and spend the day sharing what we were learning about pain and this God of ours.

Another fellow sufferer spoke of his pain that put him "on the sidelines of life." "On the sidelines," he said, "I've learned how Jesus understands our pain and holds us while we suffer." He took a strange comfort knowing our pain didn't compare to what Jesus experienced on the cross for us and how moved he was that Jesus allowed a crown of thorns to be pushed into his head. As a result of Christ's suffering, he was assured of Jesus' empathy and knew that he was always with him. The email closed with an expression of gratitude in knowing he was "not the only one who gets these headaches that no one understands." He thought (like I do) that they were a reminder that God is with us, and we need to lean on him. I suppose there is an abundance of wisdom to be found on the "sidelines of life."

Other folks who had suffered long and hard were just grateful for the reminder that God is with us. I felt our solidarity and was strengthened by it as I read their responses. I also felt a song coming on and jotted down the following lyrics as I pictured all my "new friends" enduring their pain—each in their own way—while finding a mysterious comfort in God's presence.

> I am here in purple skies. I am here in a baby's sighs. Open your eyes and you will find that I am here by your side.
>
> I am here in your pain. I am here when it rains. And when the skies clear again, we will dance together my friend.
>
> Because I love you, I do. And nothing can separate Me from you. Rest assured in my arms. I am here. I am here.
>
> I am here in your midst. I'm the praise on your lips. I'm the joy that floods your heart and I will never depart.
>
> I'm your strength. I'm your courage. I'm your shield. I'm your might. Don't lose heart. Know I'm with you in the fight.
>
> Because I love you, I do. And nothing can separate Me from you. Rest assured in my arms. I am here. I am here.

Those lyrics comfort me when I feel—like my friend in Kazakhstan—that God is distant and quiet.

Most of the readers, whether they were recommending a potential cure or sharing their own pain, closed with a sentiment that they would pray for me and my family. Can you imagine? In the midst of *their* pain, they would pray for *me*. I was humbled by their offers, moved by their compassion, and gratefully accepted their prayers. To know that complete strangers are praying for you is a comfort I can barely explain. I'm not sure how, but I know their prayers have helped. In return, I prayed for them. Misery does love company. It's hard enough to suffer. It's horrible to suffer alone. Thank God we don't have to.

One woman named Anna battled her way through a page long email wrestling with God while writing to me. I believe in the midst of her pain, she forgot who she was writing to, and I had a front row seat in the theater of her life, listening in as she struggled to understand her dilemma of pain and God. She made a positive statement about who she knew God to be and then, because of her pain, followed it up with the familiar "but then why…" query. "I know that the God that I serve is able, but I really don't understand why I have not been healed from my headaches," she wrote. Some days all she could do was "call on the precious name of Jesus for relief." Is that why God allows us to suffer so that all we can do on a given day is call on his name? Funny how desperation and pain deplete us of all resources except the ability to call out to someone outside of ourselves who has some power. I was reminded of the verse "everyone who calls on the name of the Lord will be saved."[67] That's good news for Anna and me.

Anna closed her email with a statement that to this day brings me comfort and hope: "What is so beautiful is that I know if God doesn't (heal me), I still know that He *can* and it is all just according to His will." For Anna to make that comment in the throes of her pain reflects a trust in God that goes beyond the norm—a posture of surrender that screams respect for God Almighty and whispers her great humility. I thought of Job again.

Despite the presence of God in our lives, we are obviously not immune to pain and suffering. This is not the Garden of Eden, nor is it Paradise Found. Sometimes, I think I have such a hard time with all the wrong, pain, and evil in the world because somewhere deep inside me, I know that it wasn't supposed to be like this. We weren't made for death. We weren't meant to suffer. We weren't supposed to be separated from God, left in a world that is not—at this moment—his domain. Is that why we never get comfortable with death, disease, pain, and suffering?

In the gospel of Luke, Jesus is tempted by the devil, who shows him all the kingdoms of the world in a moment of time. He says to Jesus, "To you I will give all this authority and their glory, *for it has been delivered to me*, and I give it to whom I will."[68] So we live in the enemy's domain and bad things are going to happen. The promise is that God will be with us here, and one day he will establish his domain—not just in our hearts, but everywhere. And then, he will finally reign, setting all things right—including my head.

Not long ago, I was preparing for a weekend of teaching for a spiritual retreat planned for a group of women from a Presbyterian church in New Jersey. Each year these women set aside a weekend to focus on God and their souls—a brilliant idea. The year before I had spoken to the same group and titled my talk "Trusting God"—a topic I was obviously elbow-deep in and passionate about. By the end of that weekend, I knew—if they asked me to come back—my next series of talks would be titled "Speak to Me: Hearing God's Voice." My whole "trusting God journey" had led me to a closer relationship with God—one that was more conversational than before, and I was excited to share my insights and experience with anyone who was interested.

Although I looked forward to the weekend, I was anxious for all the normal reasons. What if I went blank while speaking? What if they fell asleep during the session? What if my thoughts were incoherent and didn't materialize into anything meaningful, helpful, or true? I knew that the best way to overcome this negativity was to be as prepared as possible. So, I went to work on my outline, poured over my notes, and spent a lot of time on my knees praying for grace, wisdom, and divine intervention. I was leaving Friday afternoon, and by Tuesday, I was more than half-way through my preparations. I felt uncharacteristically under control, but early Wednesday morning I woke up with the mother of all stomach flus.

For the next three days, I was unable to get out of bed. I was so sick I couldn't even sit up and read or jot down notes. All I could do was moan and beg for mercy. The day before it hit me, my son Cole was home with the stomach flu. He had laid on the couch all day while I prepared for the weekend and occasionally checked in on him. In the afternoon, I let him watch *Batman Begins* to pass the time. While the movie was playing, I went to the family room to see how he was doing.

I sat on the arm of the couch to catch a minute of the movie and watched as the handsome Batman buckled up district attorney, love interest, and childhood friend, Rachel (played by Katie Holmes), in his super-duper, armored, indestructible Batmobile with all the bells and whistles. Rachel had just been poisoned by the bad guys and Batman was trying to get her safely to the Bat Cave where he had the antidote that would save her life. Rachel, unaware that Batman was actually her friend Bruce Wayne, was speechless, terrified, and groggy. She stared dumbfounded at the masked man, confused by whether she was in harm's way or being rescued. As he secured her seatbelt, he leaned in and stared into her eyes and slowly said, "Just trust me." In the blink of an eye, he drove off with terrifying speed, jumping off rooftops, careening through Gotham City with the frightened district attorney helpless and with no other option than to do just that—trust him. Hmm. I rubbed Cole's head of beautiful white-blonde hair, asked if he needed anything, and walked back to the study with his response of, "no thanks, mom, I'm good." Had God allowed me to see that particular clip of the movie for Batman's three words—"Just trust me"?

The following day, as I lay in bed unable to move, I was left with that particular scene playing through my head. It continued for the next three days. I couldn't believe I wasn't finished with my preparations, but, somehow, I knew God wanted me to just trust him, sit back, and enjoy the ride—kind of like Rachel. Although anxious and unprepared, there was nothing to do but lie there. So, I decided to trust that God was in the driver's seat and had me all buckled up. Each time my anxiousness surfaced, I heard him whisper, "Just trust me."

When Friday afternoon rolled around, I was almost better. I got dressed and tried to work on the computer but had no energy for it. How ridiculous to go teach a group of intelligent, vibrant women for a weekend and not be prepared. How absolutely nauseating—having nothing to do with the flu. Before I got in the car to go pick up my friend and moral support, Denise, I went to the piano to calm my spirit and clear my head. Notwithstanding my time constraints, there was a little song waiting for me. I scribbled it down quickly, sang it a few times, and felt its strength. I titled it "Surrendered" believing that waving the white flag was the key to this entire thing. It went like this:

> When I am weak, You are strong. When I have no strength to carry on, You pick me up and carry me through. And, Lord, I'm strong when I'm with You.
>
> So, go before me and lead the way. Behind me forever stay. Let Your righteous arm hold me tight, let us win the battle and this fight.
>
> Help me not forget your promises, but surrendered in Your arms, I rest.

Denise and I drove to the women's retreat with me dry-heaving out the window, hoping I would completely recover before I had to stand in front of a group of women and teach on "Hearing God's Voice." With each mile, I could hear God's soft whisper trying to comfort and encourage me. "Just trust me." Denise wondered if the women would appreciate God telling me to go and teach despite my dry-heaving. She thought dry-heaving in between teaching points might be distracting and gross and possibly discourage the women from ever wanting to hear God's voice. Her commentary made me laugh out loud. I had an unpredictable peace knowing God was in control of this mess. Such a terrifying, awful, and perfect place to be.

The retreat was held at a beautiful YMCA camp in rural upstate New York. We slowly approached our weekend accommodations, winding our way down the wooded dirt roads. We were assigned to a building named "The Castle" that stood in the distance, looking simultaneously welcoming, foreboding, and regal. Feeling like a damsel in distress, the setting was perfect. We got our things and entered "The Castle" with me looking almost as green as Princess Fiona. We were greeted by eager, earnest women who seemed happy to see us. They were anxious for a weekend full of whatever each one of their souls hoped for. I trusted I would feel fine by morning.

Despite the cozy "meet and greet" setting the women had arranged, Denise and I slipped away early, telling them we looked forward to morning and our first teaching session together. We said, "good night" and retired to our room. "God help me," I whispered as I shut the door. I could hear my new song playing over in my mind as I got ready for bed and resigned myself to the fact that I was obviously not in control.

I don't know if it was my stomach virus or the Holy Ghost, but my night was punctuated with dreams and moments of wakefulness where I was forced to open my notes and jot a few thoughts down. By morning, I felt completely well, ready, and prepared—albeit tired. As Denise and I readied ourselves for breakfast, I excitedly told her what I believed God had done in the night and how I thought he had a great morning planned for us and the women. She was relieved and promised she would keep praying.

Even though my initial outline remained the same, with my heart and ears wide open to the prompting of God, I ended each session surprised at how my talks were going. God was definitely living up to the title I gave the weekend, "Speak to Me." I felt like I had a feed in my ear as I passed along his message to the attendees. I barely touched my half-cooked notes and found myself with stories to tell, points to make, and scriptures to reference. God was faithful, and our teaching sessions were filled with his words and power. Denise and I debriefed in our room and were on our knees grateful for the fact that God was with us.

The grounds of the camp were laced with hiking trails, and on Saturday afternoon, I decided to follow one. The air was crisp, and the leaves were a brilliant red and orange. As my feet crunched up the rocky path, I realized I wouldn't be teaching at this retreat or any others if I wasn't burdened with headaches and migraines. It was obvious that my best thoughts, revelations, lessons, and stories stemmed from my pain. But more importantly, I knew I wouldn't know God to the extent that I did if my pain wasn't there to push me into his presence. On my descent, I worried about what would happen to this divine relationship if one day I actually was healed. Halfway down the mountain, I surprisingly hoped that day would never come.

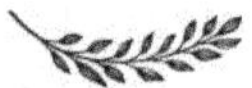

I waited patiently for the Lord; he inclined to me and heard my cry. He drew me up from the pit of destruction, out of the miry bog, and set my feet upon a rock, making my steps secure. He put a new song in my mouth, a song of praise to our God.

Psalm 40:1-3a, ESV

12

A Broken Hallelujah

Christianity teaches that … suffering is overwhelming; …suffering is real; …suffering is often unfair; but … suffering is meaningful. There is a purpose to it, and if faced rightly, it can drive us like a nail deep into the love of God and into more stability and spiritual power than you can imagine.

—Tim Keller[69]

ON THE HIKE DOWN THAT MOUNTAIN, did I really believe if God healed me from my headaches and migraines my life would be pain-free? Isn't there always more with which to contend, something else waiting in the wings of this fallen, beautiful world? Pain is all around us—broken hearts, broken bones, broken lives. There will always be something in this life causing me to reach out for help—even if God chose to heal my migraines. We have no control over the fact that pain is present, no matter its form. But we do have control over how we respond to it. Will we let it overtake us? Will we allow our pain to make us bitter, render us useless? Will we choose to live in fear because of it? Or, could we respond differently?

Reflecting on those I know living with pain, I wouldn't blame any of us if we didn't choose a different way. I think the person suffering with chronic pain, incredible loss, or any other mountain of trouble is justified if all they are able to do is curl up in a ball and sob. When my head is pounding to the point where all I am capable of is dry heaving over the edge of my bed, when the sound of air blowing through a vent is too loud, and light feels like knives cutting through my pupils, my only option is to lie down in the dark.

But even in the lying down, I have a choice. In that particular moment, I can surrender my life into the hands of a loving God and simply accept what is; or I can kick and scream, allowing my heart and mind to fill with anger, self-pity, and bitterness—an easy thing to do. But, I have found that in choosing the former my heart doesn't fill with darkness. Lying there surrendered and helpless, I simply try to wait with God until relief comes. Until he comes. For me, it's a better way.

Mike and I attended a graduation ceremony a while ago to support some of Matt's friends who were moving on to college life. We found our seats and settled in as our friend Nick, one of the community leaders addressing the crowd that day, began his remarks.

Who begins a speech to hundreds of high school seniors decked out in their caps and gowns with: "About seventy percent of you currently think, in some way, that one day you will be famous. I am here to tell you that, most likely, none of you will be." I squirmed as Nick continued. Although I suspected it was probably true, did he have to be such a buzzkill? As if it couldn't get worse, he then told the graduating class that three of his high school buddies never made it to middle age, but rather died—one from AIDS, another from a car accident, and the third from a drug overdose. The hum of the air conditioners droned awkwardly as he paused. The weight of his words filled the room.

Nick went on to expose the truth that most of us spend our lives fighting, denying, ignoring, or running from the fact that life is hard and full of pain. His encouragement and challenge to the six hundred or so teenagers was simple. In a room full of hope, a program punctuated with inspirational speeches and musical selections that made you feel like you could (and just might) become the next President of the United States, Nick challenged everyone not to run from "hard" when it came knocking on their door—which it would if it hadn't already. Instead, he implored them to embrace it. He wanted everyone to know that although we romanticize our futures, we will fare better and not be caught off guard if we expect and prepare for the hard things that are sure to happen and leverage them for growth. His plea for this graduating class was for them to process their pain, learn from it, and allow it to teach them.

Nick also suggested that we would be better off attacking "hard" and walking through the middle of it if we brought someone with some presence and power with us. Yes, you guessed it. He also found Jesus good company. Nick is one of those unique people whose passion and vulnerability leads teenagers to actually listen to him. He was able to deliver the hard truth while still fostering hope. When he was done, the room broke out in applause.

I thought how helpful it would have been to hear those words at my graduation ceremony instead of the typical "you can be anything you want to be" cheer. The ceremony ended with the class president giving his final words, and as we all filed out of the auditorium, we were glad to be reminded that "hard" has more to offer than bruises and frustration. It offers lessons that refine and grow us if, like Nick said, we process our pain.

For years, I didn't process my pain. I lived trying to ignore it, thinking I would remain unaffected if I did. Whether I was willing to acknowledge pain's presence or not, there was no changing the fact that my pain was impacting my life in some way. In finally accepting that I was a chronic pain sufferer, I had no choice but to confront it and begin finding answers to the hundreds of questions it stirred up inside of me. Pain has taken me places, introduced me to people, and taught me truths I never would have known without choosing to deal with it honestly and completely. If I didn't, I am quite sure my pain would have insidiously crept its way into every aspect of my life, filling my heart, soul, and mind with despair. In time I would have become angry and bitter—blaming God for my pain, or worse yet, deciding he didn't exist when the pain persisted, the doctors' directives failed, and my prayers for healing were denied.

My battle with pain has been fought in the ring of belief. As I have desperately gone after God and a solution to my headaches, I have landed exhausted at God's feet, still believing that he loves me, still knowing he cares. Trusting in a God of love has not saved me from my pain, but it has saved me, nonetheless.

The other morning, I met a friend for breakfast. The anniversary of her husband's unexpected death was approaching. My sympathy for her bubbled up inside when I saw her sitting at the booth waiting for me. We spent the next two hours chatting about work, kids, and whatever else came to mind. Of course, we spoke of her loneliness. Even after a year of mourning, she had no better understanding as to why God would allow her husband and the father of her children to die. Yet, she still sat in faith—bewildered and confused—choosing to believe that beauty would rise from the ashes.[70] She believed that as she and her children moved forward with each day, God would produce something good from their lives and the memory of the man they all loved. I couldn't help but notice her tears. She didn't speak those words easily and has, most likely, had to muster up courage and strength daily to believe that truth. I sat across the table from her gripping my cup of coffee filled with admiration for her faith and resolve.

That very day my friend Denise called to share a story about a family she had seen interviewed on television. Their lives were tragically changed forever after the mother's van was rear ended by a truck. Soon after they were all air lifted to the hospital, their two daughters and only son were pronounced dead. The mother and father were left to bury all of their children on a single day. I could barely listen as Denise finished the story.

Three months after the tragedy, the mother was pregnant with another baby. She said she couldn't bear the empty house and quiet. Much to their delight, they were pregnant with triplets. Yes, two girls and a boy. In the interview, the parents were careful to relay how the birth of their triplets didn't replace their other children, nor did it quench their grief, but they explained how they now had joy *added* to their sorrow.

That concept resonated with me. It's realistic. Joy co-mingled with the grief. All of it happening together in one big, tragically beautiful mess. Joy and sorrow. Pain and peace. Why do we think one can't coexist with the other when the good and the bad usually live side by side?

Soon after, I participated in another weekend women's retreat where this truth played itself out, again confirming there are two forces at work. My migraine started while driving through the foothills of the Smoky Mountains. Making my ascent to the mountain lodge hosting our event, I felt the pounding in my head intensify and began to worry about the next few days, which were supposed to be about helping others, not contending with my pain. The weekend's focus was, ironically, on healing, and I was part of the leadership team—even more ironic. If my head didn't cooperate, I knew I wouldn't be able to fulfill my role and would let the leadership team down.

Whenever I commit to doing something, I worry. I never know if a migraine will roll in and take me out of the game. I turned my music on anyway and rolled down the car windows. It was a beautiful day and no matter my thoughts, my head was out of my hands. I let my worry blow out the window along with a small piece of paper I couldn't catch before it was too late.

I arrived at the lodge excited to do my part and was greeted by the rest of the team—women filled with grace, energy, aptitude, and faith. I liked them all from the moment I met them and knew working by their side would be a pleasure. Friday night and Saturday were filled with teaching sessions, meals, and intensive spiritual homework. I was trying to be a good team member and complete my assigned jobs, but the pain in my head mounted with each passing hour. By late Saturday afternoon I knew I was done.

There was a coffee break on the schedule, and I took a moment to lie on the couch with a blanket covering my head, trying to decide what to do. Could I push through the last session, or did I need to retire to my bedroom?

Before coming to this retreat, I was told that Saturday night was the highlight. As miraculous as it sounds, many of the women attending this retreat come incredibly burdened and broken by their pasts only to get to Saturday night having experienced the supernatural grace of God. They are relieved of their shame and finally free from their misguided choices. Come Saturday evening there is cause for celebration. I was really looking forward to this part—the music, the dancing, the stories of the redeemed. I could barely wait. But there I was, retching my pain into the blanket covering my head.

I disappeared to my dark bedroom after a few of the leaders prayed for me. In my migraine fog, I remember one of them saying how she didn't know why God hadn't healed me, but she was sure his promises to me were true. I thought of one of God's promises that I cling to: "I will never leave you nor forsake you."[71] By the time I arrived at my bedroom, my mind was full of the promises of God scattered throughout the Bible. I was surprised how well I was recalling them as they marched through my brain one by one—promises of love, mercy, and goodness. I climbed to my top bunk, propped up my aching head with pillows to get as comfortable as possible and closed my eyes.

Hours passed and I could hear the women finishing up the last teaching session and heading out to the dining hall for dinner. I was alone in the lodge with my throbbing head, and the quiet was heavy. When I am left alone with my pain, I often wonder what I would do with myself if I didn't believe in God. It is desperate enough. If I didn't have my faith, if I didn't believe that God was right there with me bearing my pain, if I didn't feel his company, where would I be? I took a deep breath and muttered my usual, "help me."

I then heard the bedroom door slowly open and saw my friend Karen peering in, asking if I was hungry. I thought some food in my stomach would be good, so I climbed out of bed and shuffled over to the dining hall holding onto Karen's arm. Although my head was swimming in pain, it felt good to be out of the dark, holding onto someone.

The leadership team went straight to work after dinner, setting up the large living room for the evening of celebration. I made my way back from the dining hall and stood momentarily at the base of the staircase watching everyone get ready for the big night ahead. My sadness grew as I anticipated my climb up the stairs that led back to my bed. It was the last thing I wanted to do, and yet, under the circumstances, it seemed the only option. I grabbed the banister and closed my eyes to check and see if there was another way.

"Oh God, I want to stay downstairs for the night, but my body can't handle it. What can I do here?" I prayed.

I felt like I heard God whisper that I could do whatever I wanted—he would be with me upstairs, alone in my room, or he would be with me if I decided to stay and enjoy the party. It felt like something God would tell me—the promise of his presence while allowing me the freedom to do what I needed to do. I took a deep breath and thought about it for a minute.

But I don't know how I am going to stay downstairs with everyone while I am in so much pain. How do I do this? I thought to myself half praying, half wondering, partly whining.

Just as I finished my question, there was a phrase in the forefront of my mind— "Pick up your cross and come." I knew it was God because the thought wasn't my own. Even though I believe it is important to think about Christ and the crucifixion, it wasn't on my agenda for the night. So, I paused.

I thought about the passage in the Bible where Jesus tells those who want to follow him to pick up their cross and come.[72] What does it mean to pick up your cross? Picturing Jesus trudging up the hill to Golgotha covered in blood and sweat where he would be crucified, with crowds of people staring, screaming, and mocking him gave me a vivid picture. My cross suddenly seemed tiny and light. I released the banister and smiled. I could definitely trudge thirty feet to the couch with my migraine. Talk about perspective.

So, my aching head and I went to look for some earplugs and a place to sit. I hoped no one would pay attention to me and I would be allowed to be in the room and observe without any interaction. I stuffed the earplugs in and crawled onto a couch pushed up against the wall. The music blared, and I dry heaved into the blanket wrapped around my shoulders.

It wasn't pretty, but despite my condition, I was at the party.

With the sound muffled, I felt once removed from the moment—like a fly on the wall. I focused on everyone getting ready—the leaders and the participants—and couldn't help but smile at their apparent peace and joy. My thoughts wandered as I contemplated Jesus' words—"pick up your cross and come." That was it. When God doesn't take your pain away, what else is there to do if you don't want to lie down in the dark? The freedom to pick up my cross, my burden, my pain, and just come and not *have* to be alone in my bedroom was exactly what I needed to hear. I could come to the party anyway—feeling horrible, looking a mess, unable to sing, and incapable of dancing. I could come just the way I was and sit, watch, and listen. Even though I couldn't participate the way I wanted to or normally would have, I was able to come. I had a feeling coming would be enough. So I sat on the couch feeling surprisingly grateful and wondered what the night would look like from my sideline perch.

As the women gathered, the loud music transitioned into a soft melody. I took out my earplugs and drank in the lyrics, letting the beautiful voice sing God's spirit into every corner of my tired soul. It felt like a good long drink after a hard, long run. As the music poured out of the speakers, I felt God was near. Ironically, the song was titled, "Come In My Courts."[73] I had never heard it before and liked it immediately. The invitation to come and lay my burdens down was repeated over and over again. It was as if God himself grabbed the microphone to sing a song straight to my heart. The lyrics were sung in the first person which was even more helpful, and I did as he said. I laid down my burdens and stepped inside his courts of praise.

When the song ended, the music escalated, and I put my earplugs back in. I watched as women danced and celebrated. I noticed details I never would have had I not been relegated to the role of "spectator." To see the transformed countenances on the faces of this weekend's participants was a gift. I would never have noticed them the way I did had I not been sidelined for the night. Suddenly, I felt like the luckiest person in the room.

Watching, I realized I didn't have to open my mouth in order to sing. I didn't even have to get up and move in order to dance. All the fun of celebration could take place inside me if I acknowledged the presence of God and his spirit—which at the present moment—was hard to ignore.

While sitting there completely enjoying myself, one of the team leaders came up behind me and put the necklace she had been wearing all weekend around my neck. She told me she thought I was supposed to have it—that maybe there was something symbolic in it for me. I thanked her as she walked away and looked down to admire it. It resembled an antique door key—like one of those old-fashioned skeleton keys used back in the day when even everyday objects were pieces of art. Wrapping my hand around it, I knew it had something to do with the moment I was in, but I was too involved to figure it out. Later, I thought.

I looked out over the room, watching everyone enjoy themselves, and felt like I was going to burst—with what I don't know, but it was good. A new song started playing which was loud with a great beat. Five measures in, I could not stay seated one more second and up I went.

And, much to my surprise, there I was, dancing with a migraine.

It only lasted about sixty seconds, but it was a great sixty seconds. I don't think I will ever forget it. Coming to the party despite my circumstance proved well worth the effort—and discomfort. I was reminded how God knows how to deliver whatever it is we need and more—making it all work somehow, helping us endure, giving us what we need without necessarily changing a thing. The music ended and the women mingled before retiring for the night. I went back to my bedroom cringing in pain but filled with joy.

Once home again after the retreat, I decided to wear my new necklace until I understood what it could possibly mean for me. It didn't take long to figure it out. Really, what could be more straightforward than a key? I knew that evening at the retreat was a visible display of the many keys I've discovered to unlock the secrets in dealing with this pain of mine.

That night and my new key necklace reminded me of a few things, clarifying again that: God is with us in our pain—whether we are lying in bed or decide to "pick up our cross" and go to the party; through His Spirit, we can know joy in pain; pain doesn't necessarily have to be a negative, it can be a plus—opening our eyes and heart to more; with the pain we're given or allowed, we also have God's promises—more than I can recite, all of which are true, life giving, and good; and lastly, more often than not, the good coexists with the painful, joy mixes with sorrow. When God doesn't take our pain away, he shares it with us in a way that is helpful, comforting, transforming, and full of surprises, leaving me somehow able to accept it. When I finally took the necklace off, I was reminded that none of these keys would be in my hand unless I chose to process my pain fully and directly. Nick was right, we can either let pain destroy us or use it to learn, grow and be transformed.

There is a song that puts lyrics and melody to the coexistence of pain and glory. It's one of my favorites. My daughters, Kit and Grace, have asked me since they were little to name my favorite—my favorite color, animal, architecture, painting, person, or place. You know how kids like to play that game? But as simple as it is, I never can. It's hard to choose. I really can't name anything a favorite because it all depends. It depends on the time of year, my mood, the circumstance, the occasion, or the purpose. Naming favorites is something I just don't do—except when it comes to this song. Yes, I can honestly say Leonard Cohen's "Hallelujah" is one of my favorites.

The first time I heard "Hallelujah" was while watching the movie *Shrek* with my kids. From that moment and every time since, whenever I hear Cohen's lyrics and haunting melody pierce the air, I stop and take it in—no matter who is singing. Emotions that don't necessarily belong together stand side by side in this song. There is sadness next to hope, defeat right beside victory, and doubt coupled with resolve. It's an incredible song.

One journalist commented on the tension in Cohen's music; how his music offered the thought that nothing in this world can be reconciled. Cohen responded to the journalist's observation by saying, "this world is full of conflicts and full of things that cannot be reconciled, but there are moments when we can transcend the dualistic system and reconcile and embrace the whole mess, and that is what I mean by Hallelujah. That regardless of what the impossibility of the situation is, there is a moment when you open your mouth and you throw open your arms and you embrace the thing and you just say 'Hallelujah! Blessed is the Name.' And you can't reconcile it in any other way except in that position of total surrender, total affirmation."[74] That was it. In one breath, Mr. Cohen summed it up perfectly. I agreed completely. It is no wonder this song is one of my favorites.

I watched Cohen's live performance of "Hallelujah" in London on YouTube. He wore a suit, a fedora-like hat, and with his deep, gruff voice, drew out his "Hallelujah" into the microphone. I watched as his eyes closed and fists clenched to the music. I listened to his phrasing, made note of words he emphasized, and soaked in the author's presentation. I have heard the song sung dozens of times but never by the one who actually wrote it.

There were thousands in the audience clapping and cheering for him and the song. I wondered why it resonated so deeply with his fans. I imagined that for as many people as there were listening, there were as many reasons. That's the beauty of art—the fact that it causes a response and that each response is right—no matter what the author's intention.

I played it again and listened to the crackling "hallelujahs" in the chorus, the imperfect, desperate, feeble, and resolute "hallelujahs" in between the verses that spoke of life's spectrum. I couldn't help but compare Cohen's "Hallelujah" to Handel's "Hallelujah Chorus"–you know the one sung at Christmas time where choirs break out into, "Hallelujah, Hallelujah, Hallelujah..." and then the basses come in deep and strong with, "For the Lord God omnipotent reigneth..." The chorus ends with all parts of the choir singing at the top of their lungs, "King of Kings, and Lord of Lords..."[75] It's glorious.

Hundreds of years ago, George Frideric Handel wrote the *Hallelujah Chorus* as part of his libretto entitled, *Messiah*. In many parts of the world, it is common practice to stand during the chorus. It's been told that when Handel performed *Messiah* for King George II at the first London showing, King George rose to his feet at the onset of the Hallelujah Chorus out of respect for the "King of Kings." Royal protocol has always dictated that when a monarch rises, everyone in his or her presence must also rise. So, along with King George, the entire audience and each member of the orchestra rose to their feet as the choir proclaimed, "King of Kings, and Lord of Lords!" I get goose bumps just imagining it.

When I was in my twenties, I had the privilege of singing Handel's *Messiah* at Lincoln Center in New York City. It was a sing-along, and the auditorium was packed with sopranos, altos, tenors, and basses. We were led by professional singers and had our eyes glued to our personal copies of the *Messiah,* trying to keep pace. The notes floated and soared in the hall, and I imagined it was a taste of things to come. As we sang through the pages, the lyrics ushered us into Christ's story and the things of this world fell to the wayside. When it came time to sing the "Hallelujah Chorus," nothing else mattered but God. My spirit was called to attention as I stood before the King of Kings, humbly singing at the top of my lungs, "...and He shall reign forever and ever." What a night.

Although Cohen's "Hallelujah" and Handel's are stylistic opposites, in the end, a hallelujah is a hallelujah, no matter how you come by it or how it's expressed. I hear victory, glory, and triumph in both these songs, despite their differences.

Cohen's Hallelujah plays the chords that embrace the mess without trying to fix what cannot be fixed. It sings a melody of honesty that is simultaneously despairing and hopeful. I like this song because the messy, broken, and disappointing stand with the beautiful. The song ends in complete surrender to the truth. The truth that, regardless of our circumstance–our hurt, pain, or mess, God is worthy of our praise. Whether we see or understand all that he has done and is doing, doesn't matter. We know enough. We know him. And it is here, in this place, with our eyes transfixed on the King of Kings that we can draw our hallelujah.

For me, that kind of surrender leads to life. If I believe there is a "Lord of Song", if I believe there is a "King of Kings," I can let go of the thing—whatever it is—and trust him. It is hope and peace to me that nothing has to be resolved, fixed, healed, or understood in order to sing. Even to sing "hallelujah." I love that.

When you are someone who has asked for healing and hasn't been healed, it is important to know that a celebration can still be had and a song can still be sung. If your loved one didn't survive the wreck, you need to know that you can stand with the rest and sing despite it all. If not today, tomorrow. Though there are things we will never get over or even understand, God will help us. He will get us through. He will keep us company. He will even cause us to sing.

I have also come to realize that our lives here are just a part of our story, really just the beginning—a sample of the whole, our invitation to forever. God spends our whole lives drawing us to himself out of his great love for us. He knows our lives here are brief, and it all truly begins when we arrive at the place he is preparing for us. When I look at life through this lens—the lens of eternity—it's amazing how much more sense this all makes.

How can it be that I am not healed, but still want to lift up my voice? Why, even though my head often screams with pain, do I adore the One who created it? At the end of the day, I believe it's because I have come to know the "Lord of Song" and "King of Kings." In his presence, I am humbled and able to bend my knee in surrender. When I figuratively stand at the foot of the cross of Christ, I am overwhelmed by what God has done for me, and in that place, I am able to declare my trust and raise my hallelujah despite the pain.

I must admit my hallelujah is often Cohen's seemingly feeble and confused one, because at the end of this quest for healing, I still want to be healed. But it's a hallelujah just the same.

Along with accepting the reality of pain and yielding to God's self-restraint or higher purposes in not healing me, I also have a hope that is mostly steady. My hope lies in God, his sovereignty, and his desire to use anything and everything for his glory—including—and especially—pain. Charles H. Spurgeon, one of England's best-known preachers of the nineteenth century, wrote, "It is not hard for the Lord to turn night into day. He who sends the clouds can just as easily clear the skies. Let us be of good cheer. Let us sing Hallelujah in anticipation."[76] Our day is coming.

I know what pain has done for me, and although I would never ever choose it, there are moments when I can say I am glad it chose me. And even though I still long for my pain to go away, I know I'll be alright if it doesn't. So my hallelujah is a broken one, filled with disappointment and struggle, but it's a hallelujah nonetheless. I can sing hallelujah because God is with me in my pain, and I do not walk alone. I can stand with the choir simply because he is good, sovereign, and loves me.

Believing that God is jealous of our time and attention, believing as I do that he wants to know us, I think he often goes out of his way to catch our eye and, ultimately, capture our hearts. For me, he has done that through my pain. I don't think God has necessarily caused my pain; I just think he has chosen to use it. I can say with certainty that I wouldn't have given God my attention or time to the extent that I have if I didn't have pain in my life.

In the end, I don't know what God is up to, but I trust and love him. Through all of my pain and the measuring of pain around me, my faith *and* my doubt have led me to Jesus—who I find undeniable, despite the mess we're in. My pain and I will take this narrow road to the end where I one day hope to meet God face to face. And if my knees don't buckle and I am not rendered speechless at the mere sight of him, I might ask a few hard questions.

But if joy simply overtakes me as I see the place where pain is no more and tears are reserved solely for hard laughter, I just might slip through those pearly gates and join the celebration without a word. I hope to see you there.

> *And I heard a loud voice from the throne saying, "Behold, the dwelling place of God is with man. He will dwell with them, and they will be his people, and God himself will be with them as their God. He will wipe away every tear from their eyes, and death shall be no more, neither shall there be mourning, nor crying, nor pain anymore, for the former things have passed away."*
>
> *And he who was seated on the throne said, "Behold, I am making all things new."*
>
> Revelation 21:3-5a, ESV

Author's Note

THE COMPLETION OF THIS BOOK has been a long time coming. The manuscript was actually finished back in 2009. I know, I know. After receiving some brutal feedback from a professional editor, I was so demoralized that I just threw it in a drawer. For years.

I picked it back up again several years ago because I knew I was supposed to finish it. So, I got over myself, worked on my writing, edited some more, and threw it back in the drawer. Sharing your story, or just thinking about sharing your story, is hard.

Then in November of 2022, I was diagnosed with cancer. I thought I might be meeting God face to face and realized what a bummer it would be to meet him without completing something I knew I was supposed to do. I couldn't bear the thought and opened that drawer yet again. Even before my surgery, treatments, and all the waiting around for doctors to call, I promised myself I would get the book published before the year was out or my time was up. And here we are.

Since I finished the manuscript some time ago, I feel the need to give a bit of an update for those who wonder:

I have continued my search for a solution and tried many other treatments and potential remedies not mentioned in the book. Yes, I did the massage and Botox therapy eventually, but to no avail. I even had all my silver fillings removed in case they were the cause … and the list goes on. Sadly, I still have migraines but am happy to report that there is finally medicine available that enables me to manage them better. There's been a lot of progress in the medical world when it comes to migraines, and I no longer have to experience a 10-day episode devoid of relief—which is amazing. Also, as a result of my cancer (now in my rear-view mirror), I dove into the world of nutrition and wellness and have received added relief for my migraines there. I am grateful.

This earth is obviously not His kingdom come. That time, when all pain and suffering will cease, is coming. Meanwhile, it's good to know that God can do *greater* things than simply take our pain away. It's also good to know that we already have access to His kingdom through the Holy Spirit who is here, residing in the hearts of those who believe. Super helpful.

With that in mind, I leave you with Jesus' words:

> *Behold, I stand at the door and knock.*
> *If anyone hears my voice and opens the door,*
> *I will come in to him and eat with him, and he with me.*
>
> Revelation 3:20, ESV

Endnotes

[1] Viktor Frankl, 1905–1997, *Man's Search for Meaning*, Boston, Beacon Press, 2006.

[2] Psalm 56:8, ESV

[3] Webster's Dictionary

[4] *Hinds Feet on High Places*, p. 21

[5] *Confessions*

[6] John 8:32, ESV

[7] *The Pursuit of God*

[8] Matthew 8:2, NIV

[9] Matthew 8:3, NKJV

[10] I Corinthians 10:13, ESV

[11] Psalm 23:4, ESV

[12] Romans 8:28, ESV

[13] Psalm 46:1–7, 10–11, ESV

[14] Job 1:8, ESV

[15] Job 1:20, ESV

[16] Job 1:21, ESV

[17] Job 1:22, ESV

[18] Job 38:2–5, ESV

[19] Psalm 46:10, ESV,

[20] Proverbs 13:12a, ESV

[21] *The Secrets of the Secret Place*

[22] See Exodus 15:1–21

[23] See Joshua 4:1–8

[24] See Deuteronomy 6:7–9

[25] John 14:26, ESV

[26] Numbers 11:4–6, paraphrased by author

[27] Thomas Chisholm, 1866-1960, William Runyon, 1870-1957, "Great Is Thy Faithfulness." Hope Publishing Company.

[28] Job 1:21, CSB

[29] Matthew 6:9b–10, NKJV

[30] Robert Robinson, 1758, "Come Thou Fount of Every Blessing."

[31] Joni Earekson Tada, "Joni: An Unforgettable Story," Zondervan, 1976.

[32] See Revelation 21:1-4

[33] See Zephaniah 3:17

[34] See Jeremiah 17:14

[35] See Lamentations 3:22–23

[36] See John 6:35, Psalm 107:9

[37] See Romans 15:13

[38] *Desperate Women of the Bible: Lessons on Passion from The Bible*, Jo Kadlecek, Baker Books, 2016.

[39] John 14:13–14, ESV

[40] See Matthew 17:20–21

[41] John 16:33, NIV, emphasis added

[42] See Mark 5:24-34

[43] *Desperate Women of the Bible: Lessons on Passion from The Bible*, Jo Kadlecek, Baker Books, 2016.

[44] See Mark 2:2–11

[45] Matthew 9:2, ESV

[46] Matthew 9:6, ESV

[47] See Acts 16:25–26

[48] *Mere Christianity*, p. 149

[49] James 1:17, ESV

[50] Philippians 1:21, ESV

[51] See Exodus 33:11

[52] Romans 8:22–24a, ESV

[53] See Revelation 21:4

[54] John 5:6, ESV

[55] See James 4:8

[56] See Genesis 2:8

[57] See Genesis 12:1

[58] See Luke 2:10–12

[59] See John 19:16–42

[60] See Matthew 17:1–2

[61] See John 20:1–9

[62] See Acts 1:6–11

[63] See Acts 2:1–12

[64] See I Peter 1:8

[65] See Philippians 4:5–7

[66] See I Corinthians 13:8

[67] Romans 10:13, ESV

[68] Luke 4:6, ESV, emphasis added

[69] *Walking with God through Pain and Suffering*, 2013, pg. 30.

[70] See Isaiah 61:3

[71] Hebrews 13:5, ESV

[72] See Matthew 16:24

[73] Deluge, Album: Unshakeable, "Come In My Courts."

[74] *The Irish Times*, "Leonard Cohen: A Secular Saint" by Brian Boyd, January 28, 2012.

[75] Handel, George Frideric, 1685–1759, Messiah

[76] C. H. Spurgeon, 1834–1892

www.ingramcontent.com/pod-product-compliance
Lightning Source LLC
Chambersburg PA
CBHW031159270326
41931CB00006B/333

* 9 7 8 1 9 5 4 9 4 3 9 0 2 *